Roger Revak

For Sonam,

INTERNAL
VISION
A Ten-Day Journey
to True Happiness

I am sure
this book will benefit
you and strengthen you.
Best of wishes/prayer
Atha Rinku Sheral

Roger Revak

ISBN 10: 1-931945-98-5
ISBN 13: 978-1931945-98-1

Library of Congress Catalog Number: 2009925216

Printed in the United States of America
First Printing: April 2009

13 12 11 10 09   5 4 3 2 1

 Expert Publishing, Inc.
14314 Thrush Street NW,
Andover, MN 55304-3330
1-877-755-4966
www.expertpublishinginc.com

I was truly inspired by this man's story, not just because he survived a life-threatening brain tumor, but because of how his attitude and perspective were transformed in the process. His insightful lessons have helped me focus and regain my vision. Are you paralyzed by fear because of a shocking, life-threatening diagnosis? Has emotional pain from your childhood left you wounded, scarred, and thirsting for hope? Are you begging to be changed from a negative person to a positive person regardless of your circumstances? If the answer is yes to any of these questions, then you'll want to read this book. It's witty, thought-provoking, and easy to read. Let God touch you through Revak's inspirational message.

Kim Christianson, brain tumor survivor

You've heard the adage, "When life hands you lemons, make lemonade." Well, life has handed my brother, Roger, lemons on several occasions and he has made lemon meringue pie instead. Invariably, I've seen Roger work to turn his life trials into something positive. Turning a trial into a positive is Roger's strength. By using that strength, he discovered other natural inborn strengths. His path hasn't been easy. It was an education, an education he shares with you, so you can find your happiness. The change is real; I've witnessed Roger's transformation firsthand.

Steve Revak, Roger Revak's brother

Roger has wrapped the gift of insight in this special book for you. In these times of great challenge and change, you need to believe, make better choices, and be more focused on a daily basis. Your happiness depends on it. Choose well.

Mark LeBlanc, Small Business Success,
author of Growing Your Business!

I laughed. I cried. I loved it. This book shows transformation in its truest sense and provides guidance and methods Roger used to get through to the other side. I highly recommend this book to anyone who is facing a difficult time in their life.
Catherine Cardenuto, owner, Festive Finale

Through Roger Revak's eyes, we see his journey to find peace and true happiness within himself. I recommend this book to everyone who works in the Vision industry. This book shows appreciation for the Vision industry and reminds us of the significance of our chosen profession. It also reminds all of us, inside and outside of the vision profession, to keep our perspective on life and to laugh.
Dr. David Duff, Optometrist

This is a book with advice that can apply to anyone who has stress, anyone who doubts oneself, anyone who isn't sure of their purpose in life. Roger weaves several compelling stories of life challenges into a witty guide for the heart and soul. He provides a thought-provoking framework that coerces the reader to think deeply and honestly in order to find true happiness and self acceptance—and who couldn't use a healthy dose of both in these times? Enjoy, learn, reflect, and smile.
Beth Jett, Managing Editor, Main Anchor for KQDS-FOX 21, Duluth, MN

I have always believed true success is not something you go outside and get but rather something you go inside and become. Roger Revak shows you how to tap into that wonderful place that brings real success, significance, and true happiness. *Internal Vision* can change your life.
Craig Valentine, 1999 World Champion of Public Speaking; Founder, The Communication Factory, LLC.

As a cancer survivor, I wish I had been given Roger's book on the day I received my diagnosis. The Lessons Unlearned he provides would have made my journey so much less terrifying. However, being a survivor is not a requirement to benefit from this book. Roger's Lessons Unlearned can help us meet all of life's challenges.

Charlie Wilson, Professor of Mirth, Learning with Laughter, LLC.

Roger Revak is an extremely funny man with an extraordinarily important message. As a humorous motivational speaker and author, Roger's authentic message provides a beacon for anyone searching for true internal peace and happiness.

Dr. Lyman K. Steil; CEO and chairman, International Listening Leadership Institute; author of Effective Listening: Key to Your Success, Listening: It Can Change Your Life, *and* Listening Leaders: The Ten Golden Rules to Listen, Lead & Succeed

Roger Revak's book *Internal Vision* reveals his journey, as we identify our life trips. We all stumble, fall, and trip. Roger's story of his ability to walk on in awareness was truly a vision. Though we may not have a physical brain tumor, we all have either operable or inoperable defenses and bad habits. *Internal Vision* asks you to look at your own need to change. Roger's career as humorist and motivational speaker allows him to see the funny in the serious, which is what all of us must do to survive. *Interal Vision* will bring you to a sweeter place and one of gratitude.

Janie Jasin, speaking for over thirty years, author of The Littlest Christmas Tree

Roger Revak has turned his personal victory into a road map to success for all of us. With a story that is touching yet funny, he shares powerful lessons anyone can use to be happier and healthier. I especially like his down to earth examples. This book is both inspirational and how-to! Buy extra copies of this book and give them to the people you care about most. You'll be glad you did.

Kevin Stirtz, author of More Loyal Customers

Roger's journey will inspire, encourage, and give hope to those who are struggling with their direction in their own lives. His practical approach and simple, yet deep resounding exercises will uplift and add value to your life. He reaches to the depth of the heart when he speaks about loving oneself. *Internal Vision* is a reference text that can be used over and over to bring about happiness in one's life. I am pleased and thankful this man and this book crossed my path in life.

Paul De Baca; 8th degree Black Belt; Vice President, United States TaeKwon-Do Federation

In this era of uncertainty, it's great to have a self-help book that is easy to navigate! There are stories, examples, and learning points that are easily applicable to your current situations — whether business or personal — as long as it's about self-exploration. *Internal Vision* is practical, easy to process, and can be linked to action if change is what you seek.

Amy S. Tolbert, Ph.D., CSP, ECCO International Principal

In *Internal Vision*, Roger shares his personal story of how he viewed his medical diagnosis as an opportunity to embrace every moment of life. He provides the reader valuable tips on how to live life with an attitude of gratitude and to recognize that each day is truly a gift.

Selina Blatz, CNP, Women's Care Nurse Practitioner, Certified Health and Wellness Coach

This book is dedicated to
people who help people

Contents

Preface

One day when I was in the eleventh grade, my English teacher gave our class an assignment to write a one-page paper. We split into small groups and received feedback on our paper from other members of the group.

One of the top students in the class reviewed my paper. She said, "You have short choppy sentences, like a second grader."

I was a C minus student in high school. I had no dream, no desire, and no ability to go to college. After high school, I enlisted in the US Air Force.

After my four years in the Air Force, I returned home to a blue-collar job. Eight years later, I was laid off from the blue-collar job. After a lot of agonizing thought and, frankly, because I didn't know what else to do, I started college at age thirty.

My sophomore year I received an A on an English paper. It was the only A given to 110 students. On my paper, the professor wrote this: "You have short concise sentences, like Ernest Hemingway."

I did not share this story to convince you I write like Hemingway, nor am I implying Hemingway wrote like a second grader. Rather, I share this story to show that things aren't always as they seem. Maybe, just maybe, you have strengths you never knew you had.

When you live in the present, you discover your true self. When you discover, embrace, and nurture your true self, your hidden strengths are revealed to you. When you hone your strengths to help others, you are living your life purpose.

Introduction

This book is about discovering my self and how you can discover your self. You do not have to have a brain tumor to discover yourself — but I did.

People often asked me what I learned from my brain tumor operation. For years I could not articulate what I learned because I did not learn anything.

I unlearned an extraordinary amount. I unlearned illusions, or false self-beliefs.

You need to know my father was a verbally abusive alcoholic. He was quick-witted, sarcastic, and mean. He belittled my mother, my sister, my brother, and me. He was never physically abusive, but he could verbally slice and dice a person in half with his words. That wasn't the worst thing about Dad though. The worst thing about Dad, by far, was that he gave me his personality. When I was young, I would blurt something out without thinking and then say, "I'm sorry, I'm sorry." My dad would yell at me and say, "Quit saying things you're sorry for."

When Dad wasn't around, I would blurt out the same thing in front of my mother, and she would say, "Quit saying things like your dad."

My mother is reserved, very reserved. She is quiet and not expressive at all. From early on, I wanted to be like my mother, but I knew I was like my father. I worked hard to be like my mother. I worked hard to think before I spoke. I would get angry, without knowing why, when people did not notice how hard I was trying to be like my mother.

In high school, I worked hard to fit in. I was five feet, four inches tall, and weighed 115 pounds when I graduated from high school. I was too small for most sports, so I went out for the cross country running team. I wasn't a very fast runner, but I ran more miles than anyone else and was captain of the team when I was a senior.

I studied karate while I was an administrative clerk in the Air Force. I worked hard and was one test away from attaining my black belt when I hyper-extended my knee.

After the Air Force, I returned home to northern Minnesota and worked at a blue-collar job in an iron ore mine. I was married when I was twenty-seven years old. Three years later, I was laid off from the iron ore mine, just two months before my daughter was born.

I attended a local junior college for two years, then drove sixty-five miles, one way, the last two years to attend a university. Four years after being laid off, I graduated magna cum laude with a double major in accounting and finance. I worked hard to get those grades.

I tried to get a job close to my hometown after college, but when I couldn't get a job nearby, we moved two hundred miles away to Minneapolis.

After living in the big city for four years, I was divorced. I was thirty-eight years old.

I was angry and depressed. In fact, I was angry and/or depressed for most of my first forty years. I spent those forty years working hard to be accepted. No one knew who I really was, least of all me.

Then on the night of my fortieth birthday, I did an unusual thing. I prayed. Praying wasn't unusual for me, but this time I prayed for happiness. I was depressed, angry, and I couldn't take living that way anymore. I clasped my hands, looked up and said, "God, just give me a break for a change."

Four days after I prayed for happiness, God grabbed me by the ankles, tipped me upside down, and shook me, while I continued to whine and scream. He shook me and he shook me until all of the baggage and illusions fell to the ground.

What if you could clear your mind of your troubled thoughts?

What if you forgave yourself, and loved yourself?

What if you were really, really happy?

What if you had the courage to show the world the real you?

What if you had a gift, a purpose, to help others and yourself?

What then?

CHAPTER 1
IN THE EYES OF THE BEHOLDER

Day One
(February 8, 1996)

"Which lens can you see better through, A or B?" the optical technician asks, as she guides me through an eye test. When she is done, she says, "Your eyeglass prescription has changed." "This is my fourth prescription change in sixteen months," I explain to her, with concern. "My former eye doctor said my eyes are changing because of my age."

That's why he's my former eye doctor, I think to myself. I am not thrilled about turning forty, and I am even less thrilled about my deteriorating vision and having to wear bifocals. I've worn glasses since I was six years old, and my eyesight has been stable since then, until the last sixteen months, that is. The optical technician explains, "Our eyes go through an adjustment process at certain stages of our life. It is analogous to going over a waterfall, and hopefully, you are at the bottom of the waterfall now." As she walks out of the door with a friendly smile, she says, "The eye doctor will be in to see you in a few minutes."

Different office, same old story, I must be more assertive with this eye doctor. I must make sure he gives me a better explanation of why my eyes are changing so drastically, I think to myself. (By the way, that's who I usually think to.)

I am getting myself all worked up for a confrontation with the eye doctor before I even meet him. I am good at getting myself all worked up. I've had a lot of practice.

I am positive my allergies are somehow causing my eyes to change. I have had allergies my whole life, but they have gotten worse in the last year. My allergies give me headaches. I went to an allergist eight months ago and he gave me a skin-patch test. He prescribed an antihistamine, which I have been taking ever since. My sinus trouble and headaches are under control now. My vision is still deteriorating though, so I chose a new eye doctor from my insurance provider book at work. I am paranoid because if my eyes keep changing at this rate, I will be blind before I am fifty. I am a credit analyst for a bank, and if I can't read small print, I can't work.

Shortly after the optical technician leaves, the eye doctor walks in the exam room and introduces himself to me. He is in his early fifties and seems like a nice guy.

I must be assertive with him.

The eye doctor shines a bright light directly into my eyes, one eye at a time, and he tells me to move my eyes up and down and to the left and right. Eye doctors have given me this test dozens of times in my life, and I don't know what they are looking for, nor do I care what they are looking for. As far as I'm concerned, it is a waste of time.

When he finishes shining the light in my eyes, the eye doctor leans back in his chair, lets out a little sigh, and says, "I really don't have any good news to tell you."

What? Now, I am having trouble hearing, too.

I was sure he was going to say I don't have anything to tell you, but that's not what I heard him say. Although I am somewhat surprised by what he just said, I am also relieved because finally somebody is telling me something besides saying I'm getting old. I like this guy, he knows what the problem is and I'm sure he'll be able to prescribe something for it.

"I see a lot of edema," he says.

OK, now in addition to needing new glasses, and a hearing aide, I also need a dictionary. "What is edema?" I question, reluctantly, not wanting to admit my lack of vocabulary.

He patiently explains, "There is swelling in the blood vessels of your right eye." He then puts his right fist next to the right side of his own head and, at the same time, says, "I think there is blockage causing the swelling."

"You mean from my allergies; I knew it," I respond with a confident little giggle and a smile.

"No, not that kind of blockage," he shakes his head slightly with a serious, unnerving look on his face. "I am going to schedule an MRI for you . . . today," he says.

I don't have a clue what he's talking about, but I now know I don't like it. Even worse, I can tell by the look on his face I should be concerned. This conversation is giving me the creeps. I wipe my sweaty palms on my pant legs.

So much for first impressions, I don't like this guy anymore, and so much for being assertive. What the heck is an MRI anyway? I already feel like I flunked when I didn't know what edema was and when I guessed what was causing the blockage. I am not going to ask him what an MRI is. I think an MRI is like a CAT scan. My mother had a CAT scan a few years ago when the doctors thought she might have cancer. What is going on here?

I changed my mind. I just want my new prescription and to go home. It's about time the eye doctor tells me what's going on. But, at the same time, something tells me I really don't want to know what's going on. I don't like what he is implying even though I am not sure what he is implying.

Did I mention, I am good at getting myself worked up?

I am not a very big guy, but all of my life I have been told I have an intense look in my eyes that makes people feel uncomfortable and even afraid of me. I lean forward in my chair, smiling but with a seriously concentrated look, which is intended to make the eye doctor feel nervous. My tone has also intentionally changed. "If you are trying to scare me, it's working." I say in a threatening tone.

He rolls his chair back slightly and leans back in it. "You want me to tell you what's wrong so we can treat it properly and in a timely manner, don't you?" he asks politely.

"Yes, I'm just surprised. I don't even know what you're really talking about."

He explains the last time he saw something like this was eight years ago. He goes on to say large doses of vitamin A for long periods of time can cause swelling in the blood vessels.

That's it. I have been taking too much vitamin A, even though I haven't been taking it for long.

I read that vitamin A is good for the eyes. I thought vitamin A would stop my eyesight from deteriorating, so for about a month I've been taking the maximum recommended dosage (maybe even a little more). It's my fault for taking too much vitamin A. Now I'm calming down a little; he had me scared for a minute.

He doesn't know I am calmer now, so he tries to calm me down some more, "If it makes you feel better, I'll ask another doctor to come in and give his opinion without telling him what I think it is."

What the heck, might as well. I nod my head and say, "Sure."

The eye doctor leaves the room, and after a few minutes, he returns with a second eye doctor. The second eye doctor looks like a no-nonsense, serious guy, also in his fifties. He takes his turn shining the light in my eyes and says there is swelling in both eyes, but the right eye is worse. He asks me if I've had any problems lately.

I tell both eye doctors about all of my recent prescription changes and also about the fog in front of my right eye. For the last week or so, I have had a fog in front of my right eye, but only when I wake up in the morning. I splash a little water in my face and the fog goes away.

I am sure the fog must have something to do with my amblyopia (lazy eye). When I was six years old, I had to wear a patch over my left eye because I was practically blind in my right eye. My eyesight in my right eye improved after wearing the patch over my left eye because it strengthened my right eye. Now, with glasses, my vision is corrected to 20/20 in both eyes, until my prescription changes again, that is.

The two eye doctors turn away from me and began discussing when the MRI needs to be scheduled.

This gesture of turning away from me and talking about me as if I'm not here is very irritating. I am already on edge, and this discussion they are having about me, right in front of me, makes me feel even more anxious.

Let's face it, I'm scared, and I can tell both eye doctors think there is something wrong other than too much vitamin A.

I interrupt them, point at the first eye doctor and say, "You are scaring me," and then I turn to the second eye doctor and say, "And you are telling me you agree with him, right?" I ask this very assertively, not aggressively (my opinion, of course, not theirs).

The second eye doctor tries to calm me down by saying, "We just want to have you tested so we can rule out the worst thing first." He then leaves after a brief discussion with the first eye doctor.

The first eye doctor comes over, sits down by me again, and calmly says, "I understand how you feel."

Big mistake! My body tightens as I get set to yell at him and ask him how he can possibly know how I feel.

Before I get a chance, he brushes his hair back and shows me a four-inch scar on the top of his head. "I had a brain tumor six years ago," he tells me.

He finally said it. What . . . Arrrrrgh! I grit my teeth and put my head down. I look up suddenly and uncontrollably blurt out, "Are brain tumors common or what?"

This is unreal. I can't believe he's telling me I might have a brain tumor, and I can't believe he's had one. This must be a nightmare. I am ready to wake up now.

Then he says, "I am going to give you a field vision test to check your peripheral vision. Before that, though, I will tell the secretary to schedule you for an MRI today."

After the field vision test, the eye doctor shows me the results, which indicate the peripheral vision in my right eye isn't very good. He then says, "It's four o' clock now. Your MRI appointment is at 5:30 this afternoon. I'll call there later tonight and try to find out the results."

"You better call there at 5:30 to see if I show up," I laugh, but I am not kidding. I can't believe I am not going to wake up from this nightmare.

As I leave the eye doctor's office, and get into my car, I am a bit numb and in disbelief as I drive to get something to eat before going to the hospital for my MRI. Even though I have never experienced a real state of shock before, I know I must be in shock.

As I am driving to get something to eat, I start talking out loud to myself.

"So much for my plan to be assertive with the eye doctor, and so much for going back to work this afternoon." I have a work deadline I have to meet by tomorrow, but all of a sudden it doesn't seem to bother me as much as it did earlier in the day.

I'll take responsibility for not meeting the deadline at work but I am not going to tell anyone about this.

My biggest fear in the whole world is being called stupid and being laughed at. Dad called me stupid more often than he called me by my name when I was young. Kids in school picked on me when I was young because I was one of the smallest kids in the class. I have spent my whole life trying to avoid criticism and looking for acceptance. I have spent my whole life trying to avoid situations like this one.

Even though I am scared, for some reason I find this whole situation somewhat funny and ironic because this morning, before I went to the eye doctor, I thought

I had a lot of problems. Now I can't recall having any problems before going to the eye doctor.

I thought I reached the bottom after being laid off, going to college, moving, and getting divorced. Now, I might have a brain tumor. Maybe there is no bottom at the end of my life's waterfall.

Five years ago I was married, living in my small hometown with lots of friends and relatives nearby. Five years ago, my father passed away. Four years ago, I moved to Minneapolis to find a job and start a new career. Two years ago I was separated and a year ago the divorce was final. Last year my mother moved away to Idaho to live by my sister, Linda. My brother, Steve, lives in Nebraska. The only relative I have in Minnesota is my nine-year-old daughter, Alissa, who lives with her mother, except every other weekend when she stays with me. I don't have any long-term friends in the area, only my co-workers and a few married friends whom I don't see very often.

After all of the changes, I thought I was at the bottom of my life's waterfall. I thought my life would start getting better — until this eye doctor appointment.

"This eye doctor must be crazy," I say out loud to myself, shaking my head. I'm sure eventually I will find out everything is OK and the doctors will yell at me for taking too much vitamin A. Then, of course, I will beat myself up for being stupid, like I always do, and everything will be all right. I'll be embarrassed about this later — but my adrenaline sure is flowing now.

I park my car in the hospital parking lot, and begin to walk towards the hospital. As I walk, my thoughts of the eye doctor appointment and the future MRI appointment disappear.

I am walking. I am looking at the blue sky and a few clouds. I am listening to cars go by and people talking. I feel the cold of a February day in Minnesota. I am right here right now. That is all I know for sure.

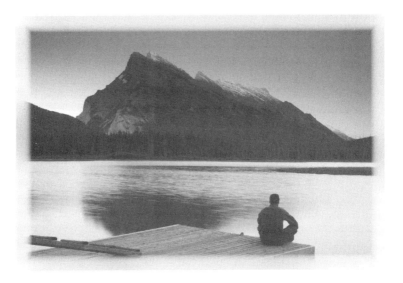

Lesson Unlearned #1
What does living in the present mean?

You are living in the present when you focus all your energy on what you are doing right now. There are three distinctive characteristics to living in the present.

1. Your external awareness becomes razor sharp. You are aware of everything going on around you. You are aware of your breathing and all of your senses are on high alert. You are not concentrating on any one of your senses more than the others.

2. Your internal awareness is also sharp. You are aware of all of your own feelings and thoughts.

3. After all of the thoughts float by, there is silence, and energy appears. Depending on the situation, the energy may give you peaceful joy, it may give you intuition and answers, or it may make a difficult physical activity seem effortless.

Common places where people experience being present are:

1. while meditating or praying

2. while working out

3. when fully engaged in something they love to do

4. while being alone in nature

5. when watching a child play or playing with a child

6. when they were babies

7. when a doctor tells them they might have a brain tumor or some other shocking diagnosis.

These are examples of common present-moment experiences. Newborn babies are present because their minds have not yet developed to stop them from being present. Since we all were newborn babies, we have all been present. We can live in the present any time we choose, we just have to remember how to live in the present and practice. With practice we become more aware and get better.

Some people believe present-moment experiences are an escape from reality. The truth is the present is *REALITY*. Anytime you are not in the present, you are in an illusion created by your own mind. It might be a productive and positive illusion or a detrimental and negative illusion. Either way, it is an illusion.

Here are a few more truths and fallacies about living in the present.

1. Living in the present means you are going to sell all of your worldly possessions, meditate all day

long, and travel around the world because you do not believe in living for the future. False. Living in the present simply means you concentrate on your present activities including breathing, seeing, hearing, smelling, tasting, and touching.

2. You cannot have goals and live in the present. False. You still have goals in your conscious and subconscious mind, but you realize your mind is not reality. Your conscious mind chooses your destination, your subconscious mind plots the path, and you concentrate all your energy on experiencing the path in the present.

3. Living in the present is referred to by some as being awake and some refer to it as being enlightened. True. But it's not that big of a deal. Being enlightened just means you have the perspective not to take your thoughts too seriously.

4. Once you are enlightened, you are present all of the time. False. You should not strive to be present all of the time; otherwise you would be like a newborn baby, but you can learn to be present when you want to be.

Now that you have a better understanding of what it means to be present, start to notice those times when you are present. Look for opportunities to be present. Give yourself credit each time you practice living in the present, no matter how long or short the experience.

Let's continue on with the first day of my journey.

CHAPTER 2
GOING TO
THE MOON

It is six o'clock in the evening, and I'm at the hospital watching a video about MRIs with an elderly woman, who is also waiting to have an MRI. This video is for people who have not had an MRI before, and it is narrated by an astronaut who summarizes the video by saying, "I'm sure you're feeling a little anxiety right now, but remember I felt anxiety when I first went to the moon; it's only natural."

I turn to the elderly lady and ask, "So, is an MRI just like going to the moon?"

She responds with a friendly smile, "I don't think it's the MRI that causes anxiety, son. I think it's the results of the MRI that cause anxiety." She then asks, "Why are you having an MRI?"

I smile back and respond, "My former eye doctor thinks my eyes are changing because I'm getting old, and my new eye doctor thinks my eyes are changing because I have a brain tumor. I think I like my former eye doctor better."

After the video, the nurse calls the elderly woman in for her MRI and later, when she is done, I hear the nurse tell the elderly woman they will notify her of the results in two days.

Two days! I have to wait two full days to find out the results. I'm sure the results will turn out to be OK, but I'll give myself an ulcer while I'm waiting for them.

A little while later, the nurse comes back into the room, calls out my name, and I go into the examining room. She asks me to lay flat on my back and be still.

The MRI is a tube-shaped cylinder, and it reminds me of a culvert. I remember when I was a kid my friends and I would crawl through a culvert in the road, then laugh while cars drove over us.

I lie flat on my back with my eyes closed. It feels like I am lying in a cave while tiny jack hammers are pounding away on the outside. I wish I could go to sleep in here. Then I would wake up in my bed and find out this is all a nightmare.

As I am getting out of the MRI cylinder, the technician tells me I have a phone call.

A phone call?

"Now I know it's a bad dream. No one knows I am here," I say, laughing nervously at the technician.

"It's your eye doctor," she says with a polite smile.

I take the phone, and listen as the eye doctor explains the MRI pictures are going to be sent to a radiologist right now. The eye doctor then says he will call a neurologist and ask him to confer with the radiologist.

"If you don't mind waiting for forty-five minutes, I'll ask the neurologist to call you," the eye doctor says.

I can tell my mind is starting to go numb again, as I respond, "Sounds good; thanks for keeping me so informed. So does this mean there is a tumor?" I ask this question as a formality, out of instinct, with no emotion, because the truth is I don't want to know the answer.

"There's something there; we don't know what it is yet. It's out of my field of expertise now, but I'll have the neurologist call you," he answers politely.

I can't argue with logic anymore. I can't believe this is happening, but I can't deny what is going on here. So much for my vitamin A theory; I don't think the eye doctor would be asking the neurologist to call me at 7:30 at night if I was taking too much vitamin A.

As I wait for the neurologist to call, the blankness in my mind and the numbness in my body increases with each breath. Nothing could make me happy right now and nothing could make me sad. My mind is blank and my body is numb.

Thirty-two minutes after I am done talking to the eye doctor, the technician tells me I have a phone call from the neurologist. The neurologist introduces himself and tells me I should call his secretary tomorrow at

9:00 a.m. to schedule an appointment, which will also be for tomorrow.

I don't have too much to say right now, but I manage to gather my thoughts slightly and ask the neurologist, "Does this mean there is a tumor, and if there is, what's next?"

The neurologist explains he has not yet seen the results of the MRI. He has only conferred with the radiologist. He will have the results sent to his office in the morning and discuss them with me tomorrow after I call his secretary for an appointment.

I'm not used to getting so much attention; it makes me feel kind of important. This is just like winning the lottery — only the opposite.

I am pleased the doctor has discovered what is wrong, but I am very afraid. I have felt fear before, but never like this. This fear is much more intense, but it is not only the intensity of the fear that sets it apart from past fear in my life. This time I am afraid of something bigger than avoiding my own anxiety. This time I am afraid of something real.

Lesson Unlearned #2
What is fear?

There are two kinds of fear: rational fear and irrational fear. Rational fear protects us from harm. A fear becomes irrational when your behavior to avoid the harm is no longer logical. You are fearful of potential harm, and also fearful of the thought of harm, which triggers a negative emotion. Examples of negative emotions are anger, guilt, and resentment. You become fearful of your own thoughts and significantly alter your behavior to avoid negative emotion.

Part of our subconscious mind keeps track of past positive emotional experiences, which are triggered by outside stimulus. For my purposes here, I will call this part of the subconscious mind the ego. The ego also keeps track of past negative emotional experiences. The ego tries to avoid similar future negative emotional experiences.

I learned at a young age that criticism towards my natural, quick-witted comments, my natural facial expressions, and gestures stirred negative emotions in me. Since I did not have many positive emotional experiences in my childhood, I concentrated on avoiding experiences that triggered negative emotions. I was afraid to do anything that would hurt someone or cause someone to tease me and pick on me.

My fear of criticism was so deeply ingrained inside of me, I thought it was part of my innate personality. I assumed I was cursed with a bad personality from my father.

My fear of criticism kept me from taking chances and from taking on responsibility because I did not see any benefit in taking chances or taking responsibility. I only saw potential for more anxiety. My fear of criticism also kept me from having a life dream. Do you have a dream? If not, why not? If the reason you do not have a dream is because of fear, you can unlearn fear and start to dream.

I wanted to be accepted by others and I wanted to avoid criticism. I did whatever I could to be accepted and to avoid criticism. Of course, I wasn't aware I was doing this.

How do we discover irrational fear and see it for what it really is — an illusion created by our own mind?

Rational fear scares irrational fear away because rational fear exposes irrational fear's cowardice.

- One way to discover irrational fear is to compare it to rational fear. Close your eyes and imagine a grizzly bear is chasing you through the woods. Your thoughts and your visualization can create the same terrifying emotions as if your imagination were reality. The only difference is when you open your eyes, there are no real bear claws and teeth to contend with. The fear of the bear was an illusion created by your own mind. With thought and visualization, your mind creates visual scenes, which connect to emotions, but there is no real present danger. The danger is your mind creating a dramatic illusion.

When you experience rational fear, there is real present danger.

How can you tell the difference between a dramatic illusion and real present danger?

Think about your fears and where each one originated. Then consider how real your danger is right now. Whenever you feel your fear arise, ask yourself if there is real present danger right now, or if your mind is projecting past emotional trauma into the future. Keep working at this and you will succeed in learning, knowing, and living the fact that irrational fear cannot survive in the present. Now you know what living in the present is and you know irrational fear does not exist in the present.

Let's get back to the story and learn how to be present.

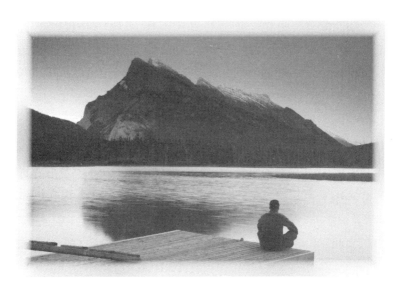

CHAPTER 3
HOW WAS YOUR DAY?

The clock on the wall in the hallway shows it is seven o'clock as I walk out of the hospital at night after the MRI. I walk past a janitor who is mopping the floor of an otherwise empty hallway. The janitor says, "Hi, how's it going, man?"

I instinctively say, "Good," as I walk by him. Then I stop, as if I have been suddenly woken up from a deep sleep. I turn, look directly at the janitor, and wait for him to look back at me. Then, with a smile, I say, "I went to the eye doctor this afternoon for a routine check-up, and now I am walking out of the hospital knowing I have a brain tumor."

The janitor drops his mop to the floor, stares at me, and responds in a quiet voice, "I'm sorry, man." Then with a semi-shocked look on his face, he stoops down to pick up his mop.

I turn to walk away, smile to myself, and think, I bet it will be a long time before he asks another stranger, "How's it going?"

As I get into my car and begin driving home, I cannot help but wonder what is going on. The eye doctor is going out of his way for me, and I sure appreciate it, but it scares me.

I am forty years old. I assumed I would live to be at least seventy. Dad lived to be seventy-two, and he never met a cigarette or a drink he didn't like. There is one good thing about this, though. I can't blame myself for this. I don't think anybody would ever blame me for causing this, except for Dad, that is.

My dad drank alcohol from the day I was born until the day he died. I am the youngest of three children. My sister is six years older than I am and my brother is three years older than I am. I have been told Dad started drinking heavily shortly after I was born, but I don't know why. I wasn't sure he was an alcoholic until I was nineteen years old. I had a drug and alcohol class one day when I was in basic training in the Air Force, and someone asked the instructor, "What if somebody drinks steadily all day, but never gets drunk?" The instructor replied, "He or she is drunk all of the time; you just don't know it because you've never seen him or her sober."

That was my dad, never sober.

I had a four point zero grade point average during my first two years of college. Just before I received my two-year associate degree I went to my parent's house and told my dad I was at the top my class out of eight hundred students.

He was reading the paper, having a drink, and smoking a cigarette. He took a puff of his cigarette, looked up at me, and said, "There must be a lot of stupid people going to that school." Then he went back to reading the paper, finishing his drink, and smoking his cigarette without another word.

That was my dad, never sober and always sarcastic.

I want to be like my mother and my brother. They are so quiet, reserved, and nice. My mother and my brother do not say things to hurt anyone and no one criticizes them for saying the wrong thing. Instead, I blurt stuff out that I often regret.

I have spent most of my life trying to change to please other people. I have read dozens of self-help books, gone to counseling, and even attended a few Adult Children of Alcoholics meetings. I do everything I can to *not* be like my dad. I get mad at myself when I screw up, and I get mad at others when they do not notice how hard I am trying not to blurt stuff out.

This brain tumor thing changes everything, though. My life-long issue of having a not-so-delightful personality may have to take a back seat because I might have a real problem now.

As soon as I enter my apartment, I walk straight to the phone and call my brother, Steve. After he tells me about his day, I tell him about mine, and then I say, "A brain tumor, it's like a bomb. What could be worse than a brain tumor?"

"Hey, it's not testicular cancer," my brother says cheerfully.

"Good point," I laugh. Maybe my brother does have a little bit of Dad in him.

Next, I call a new-found woman friend, who happens to be a nurse. I tell her the story and then ask her, "Do you think I made it up?"

"No," she says, "Not even you would make this up."

I laugh, and then say, "You're right, if I made it up I would have told you it's testicular cancer."

She reminds me of our conversation the night before when it was my idea to exchange thoughts on our spiritual beliefs. "It's almost as though you knew something was going to happen," she says.

"I don't think so," I respond, adamantly. "I would have never guessed this in a million years, and I still don't believe it. I'm sure it will be all cleared up tomorrow."

Then she asks, "What is your new eye doctor's name?"

"I don't know; I can't remember."

"Roger, this guy might have saved your life, and you don't even remember his name."

"Once I remember it, I'll never forget it. How's that?" As soon as I hang up the phone, I look up the eye doctor's name in my insurance provider book.

As I lay in bed I began to pray, just as I do every night. Most people who know me would not believe I pray every night because I haven't gone to church in years, but spirituality is very important to me. I was thirty years old when I was finally able to articulate my spiritual beliefs. Before then, I felt like I was being pulled in all kinds of different directions. Once I finally figured out what I believe, people quit asking me what I believe.

My personal beliefs are based on one declarative statement: There is a God. I believe if I was all alone, with nobody around to influence me, I would declare there is a Higher Power who created this universe. For lack of a better term, I call this Higher Power "God."

My belief in a Higher Power is my one and only leap of faith. I believe mankind has the ability to teach each other about math, music, kindness, and all other subjects except God. I believe the only way for me to have a relationship with God is through personal prayer. I am skeptical of situations where God has communicated through a few chosen people, especially when God tells those people that other people should give them money in the name of God.

Rather than pick and choose which interpretation of God's word is correct, I choose not to listen to anybody else's view, or read anything regarding third-party opinions about God.

I pray. I talk with God and I believe he listens.

I have never met anyone who believes what I believe, and I have never tried to convert anyone. We are a congregation of one. Membership isn't growing, but it is stable — as long as I live, that is.

I do not have answers to why we are here, how things happen, why things happen, or what happens after we are dead. When it comes to God and the Universe, I accept and trust the unknown. It's a mystery to me, and I am OK with that.

Some people think I am an atheist or an agnostic, but I am not. Some people think because my beliefs are so simple, they are not strong, but my faith is very strong. Then, again, my faith has never been tested like it may be tomorrow.

Lesson Unlearned #3
How do you live in the present?

Being present is not about your religious beliefs. With regards to being present, your religious preference does not matter. To be truly present, though, one must be fully grateful for this moment. If you do not believe in God, then be thankful for life itself.

When you are in the present, you appreciate *everything* **about this moment.** All of your energy is concentrated on activity, and you are grateful for the activity.

There is no past to limit you and no future to worry about. There is no thought and no mind to stop the flow of energy. You simply concentrate on experiencing and appreciating the activity of this moment.

There are no judgments, labels, or expectations. Imagine a baby who is walking for the first time. The baby doesn't say to himself or herself, I am doing a good job or bad job of walking. This is fun, or this isn't fun. The baby just concentrates completely on the activity of walking, and when the activity is over, the baby says to himself or herself, Wow!

Here is an exercise for you.

Take a breath. Appreciate the fact you can breathe. Wiggle your fingers and your toes. Appreciate the fact you can move your fingers and toes. Take another breath. Look out the window. Appreciate the fact you can see. Take another breath. Listen, just listen. Appreciate the fact you can hear. Take another breath. Smell the air. Appreciate the fact you can smell. Take another breath. Lick your lips, and bite your tongue. Appreciate the fact you can taste and feel. Take another breath. Now appreciate all of your senses at the same time.

Congratulations, you are present — in the activity of the moment. Now you know what being present is. You know that irrational fear doesn't exist in the present and you know how to be present.

Next is Day Two of my journey to true happiness.

CHAPTER 4
AND THEN ALL OF MY PROBLEMS WERE GONE
Day Two

I called the neurologist's office at nine o'clock on Friday morning to schedule my appointment for 9:30 (one half hour later).

My legs are shaking and my palms are sweating as I walk into the neurologist's office. I introduce myself to the neurologist, and he gives me a confused look back. Then he says, "Oh, yeah, you need to go down the hall to the neurosurgeon's office."

It is a short distance and a long walk to the neurosurgeon's office. I introduce myself with a nervous smile on my face and a lump in my throat. The neurosurgeon stands up and shakes my sweating hand. He is about forty-five years old and seems like a pleasant man. We talk for a few minutes about our lives. I tell him I am divorced and I have a nine-year-old daughter. After we're done with the introductions, he says, "Let's go take a look at it."

We walk into the hallway where there are pictures from the results of the MRI hanging on the wall. My throat is dry and my eyes are watering. I have difficulty focusing as I look at the pictures.

Oh, my God. Ohhhhhhhhh, my God.

Roger C. Revak
MRI scan – head
February 8, 1996

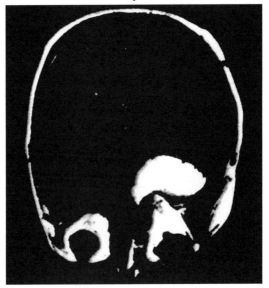

It does not take the training of a radiologist or a neurosurgeon to tell there is something wrong with this picture.

Yesterday was shocking. Today is terrifying. There is a ball behind my eye. I would give anything for this not to be real, but I am staring at reality and reality is staring back at me.

How ironic it is. Yesterday the eye doctor put his fist next to the side of his head to describe the blockage. That is how large the tumor appears to be, the size of the eye doctor's fist.

"It looks big," I mutter in a trembling voice. "Is it large compared to what you are used to seeing?" I ask in disbelief.

"It's large," the surgeon responds, "it's about the size of a small peach. That may be the good news. If something this size were dropped into your head right now, you would be dead. In order for your brain to adapt to this, the tumor must have grown very slow. I think there is a 99 percent chance it is benign, non cancerous."

"How long do you think it has been in there?" I ask in a humble tone.

"I think it has been there a long time. I think it has possibly been there for twenty years," he answers.

Twenty years! I wonder how many people will say, "I knew he was crazy ten years ago." I have struggled most of my life to be accepted and to prove I am normal. Now I am staring at the unarguable evidence that proves I am not normal.

"It looks like it might be wrapped around the optic nerve. That might be a problem when I go to take it out," the surgeon informs me.

"So worst case scenario, I go blind in one eye?" I ask optimistically, because given the situation, I don't think I would miss my right eye.

"No," he says, "worst case scenario, you're dead."

"I knew that," I chuckle, knowing it is not his job to support my impossible hopes, but wishing it was.

The neurosurgeon continues. "Worst case scenario, you won't survive the operation and there is a possibility you will suffer a stroke during the operation. But if we don't operate soon, the tumor will burst, and when it does, your daughter will lose her father for sure."

I like it when people come right out and tell me the way it is. I don't like it when people beat around the bush, and I don't like it when they butter up the truth. But honestly, I've had my fill of straightforwardness in the last two days.

The fear has taken over my whole body and has replaced all of my emotions. I am not sad, depressed, or angry. I am scared to death — of death.

I must have a look on my face like I am going to run away because the surgeon adds, "The worst thing you could do is nothing. The tumor is so big it is going to rupture soon. We don't have to operate today, but we can't wait long. Today is Friday, I've scheduled you to arrive at the hospital next Tuesday, and I will operate on Thursday," he says.

Immediately, I blurt out with a laugh, "You're not going out drinking Wednesday night, are you?"

"No," he responds, looking at me peculiarly, smiling and shaking his head.

As I stare at the picture on the wall, I have no hopes, no dreams, and no expectations. I have my sense of humor. I am possessed by a spontaneous wit. I cannot help but laugh at myself and the world. I have always had a natural ability to be witty, but, of course, my mouth has gotten me in trouble. I try to suppress my quick wit for fear of saying something wrong, saying something that might hurt someone's feelings, or saying something that might give someone a reason to criticize me.

I know some people will say my sense of humor is a way of coping with this situation. But the truth is I have been coping by suppressing my sense of humor to avoid conflict with others for most of my life. My coping skills may have avoided some conflict with others, but suppressing my real personality has caused internal conflict.

There is no internal conflict now.

I have no fear of being accepted or being rejected, and no guilt. The only fear I have now comes from the picture on the wall. The reality of the tumor has put my irrational fears in perspective. The reality of the tumor has unlocked the door, which has imprisoned my spirit and now my spirit has kicked the door open. I may not live through this, but I am definitely alive now. I can feel it. Perhaps for the first time, as long as I can remember, I feel alive.

In addition to my sense of humor, I have a heightened sense of awareness to detail, and I have a newfound, uncanny ability to look at something intensely, so intensely I can permanently engrave it into my memory. I am driven by this keen sense of awareness because I do not want to miss or forget anything.

We walk back into the neurosurgeon's office, and the neurosurgeon begins writing something down. As he is writing, he reminds me there is a possibility I may have a stroke during the operation. If this happens, I will lose the sight in my right eye, and the left side of my body will be paralyzed. He explains I may also have a seizure, and he gives me a handwritten prescription for anti-seizure medication and another prescription for steroids. In addition, he tells me it may not be possible to remove the whole tumor. If this happens, he will either operate again or treat the remaining portion of the tumor with radiation. He explains the surgery will be extensive and last eight hours.

"How many do you have scheduled for next Thursday?" I ask.

"Only one," he responds politely with a smile. He goes on to tell me he will go in through the top of my head, above my right eye. He doesn't tell me how he will get into my skull, and I don't ask.

I'm preoccupied with the picture of the tumor; I don't care how he gets it out, as long as he gets it out. Pain is not only a foregone conclusion, it is a positive scenario considering the alternatives.

He explains the plan for next week to me. "You are scheduled to be admitted into the hospital and have an angiogram on Tuesday. You will have an embolization on Wednesday, and I will operate on Thursday."

I have heard of an angiogram before, but I don't know what it is and what is an embolization? I am blown away right now; I don't even ask.

As I walk out of the surgeon's office and start to drive back to work. I start to talk out loud to myself again. "I don't know which is worse, the fact there's a baseball in my head or the fact there is room for a baseball in my head. I am obviously not normal. A normal person would be dead already!" I crack myself up.

Laughter is the best medicine,
next to laser surgery that is.

I'm so scared, but yet I've never been so uninhibited. I am focused and my sense of humor is in charge. Well, one thing is for sure, if I was depressed before, I am not depressed any longer.

For me, depression is a luxury,
a luxury financed by time.
Without time I cannot afford
to be depressed.

I am focused on making the most of every trivial minute because there are no trivial minutes any more. I am so focused on living; nothing on earth scares me. Don't get me wrong, I am plenty scared, but not of anything on earth.

Back at work, I tell my supervisor the results of my doctor's visit, which I had informed him about in the morning before I left work. He tells me the president and the CEO want to talk with me. The two of us go into the CEO's office and the CEO tells me that it is in my best interest and the best interest of the company if I take the rest of the day off and also Monday.

I laugh to myself because I can see his point about why it may be slightly disruptive to the workplace if anybody asks me, "How's it going?"

The president tells me he will notify the rest of the employees of my situation in a company memo. They all shake my hand and wish me good luck and a speedy recovery. Nobody mentions today's work deadline that seemed like the most important thing in the world yesterday.

Back at my apartment, I sit on the couch in my living room. I am overwhelmed with emotions. I look up in the air and shake both of my fists, as I yell out loud, "How could you do this to me? You dirty rotten!"

Then I realize I might actually meet God next Thursday. I laugh at my self. I laugh at my self until I cry.

Afterwards, I try to relax as I sit on the couch and watch a daytime talk show. There is a guru as a guest on the show, and he is describing his new book and how he can teach anyone to become enlightened and relinquish all of their problems if they will only buy his book for thirty dollars and follow his strict guidelines.

Bored with the show, I stand up and look out of my picture window at the snow covered courtyard below. I notice a squirrel rummaging at the base of a nearby tree. The squirrel looks so content and yet so aware of everything as it looks around for danger. Then, for some reason, it decides to take off and run across the road.

Unfortunately, there is car zooming down the road at the same time. The squirrel stops in the middle of the road, looks directly at the car, and then instinctively runs back to side of the road and continues up a tree to safety. While in the tree, the squirrel turns towards me and looks directly at me. I see a combination of fear and excitement in its eyes. I can practically see the adrenaline rushing through its pounding little body, for the squirrel may not be smart enough to keep from running in front of a car, but it's smart enough to know it's lucky to still be alive. I swear, the squirrel winks at me and continues up the tree to live out the rest of its hopefully less eventful day.

I pick up my notepad and write what I just learned from my new guru, the squirrel.

ENLIGHTENMENT

Every creature innately knows that time on earth is limited and the length of its own life is unknown. Only mankind has the arrogance to ignore this universal fact. Every creature has an obligation to survive, even though all efforts will be futile in the end. Acceptance of the inevitable end combined with the struggle to defer it creates a sharp, present-moment awareness.

This consciousness automatically creates an unintentional by-product referred to by the ignorant as enlightenment. But, for the enlightened creatures, there is no leisure time to gloat, bask, or even be attached to one's own life. For whether they are blessed or cursed, these creatures have already painfully felt and grieved their own imminent death. Now they laugh back at mankind with the knowledge that the highest form of enlightenment is simply living each extra moment.

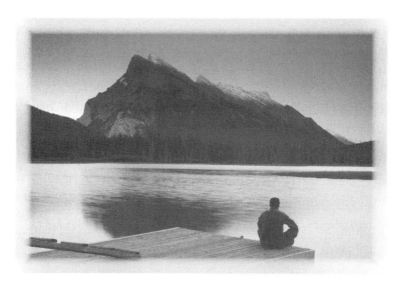

Lesson Unlearned #4
What's In It For Me?

Advantages of living in the present include:

1. **When you concentrate on your present activity, you take responsibility for your actions.** By concentrating on your present activities including breathing, seeing, hearing, smelling, tasting, and touching, you are concentrating on what you can control. Whether you are sitting down or climbing a mountain, you are taking responsibility for your actions.

2. **There is less stress in the present because you are concentrating on what you can control.** There is stress when you concentrate on the past because you cannot change what happened in the past. There is stress in the future because you cannot control everything in the future. When you focus on your present actions, you do not sabotage your present actions by focusing on something else.

3. **When you live in the present you have more energy.** When you immerse yourself into your present activity, you experience what athletes call "the zone." The zone is an effortless feeling.

You do not have to be an athlete to experience the zone. The feeling of being in the zone is a result of concentrating fully on the activity and not caring about the outcome of the activity. When you concentrate so intensely on the activity, your mind becomes silent and there is extra energy. The zone is a result of unconditional love for the activity. There is no pressure when you are in the zone because there is no expectation of the outcome of the activity.

Have you ever had an experience where you worked real hard at something because you wanted the outcome so badly, but you couldn't get it because you put too much pressure on yourself to achieve an outcome? Then you finally gave up. You got to a point where you didn't care any more about the outcome, and you accomplished your goal. It felt like you didn't even try. You got what you were striving for, but not until you gave up wanting it. You took pressure off of yourself by giving up your future expectation and just experiencing your present activity to your fullest potential. This doesn't mean you shouldn't have a goal, it simply means you concentrate on the path to the goal instead of the goal.

4. **When you are present, you are aware, not only of your actions, but also of your thoughts.** You are aware of your self-talk. Self-talk is similar to computer output. Whatever outside input is put into your subconscious mind, it comes back to you in the form of self-talk. If your self-talk is negative, it is because the input was negative.

5. **You distinguish between your self-talk and your intuition.** Intuition is a feeling that is not based on any outside influence or past experience.

6. **When you are present, you experience and appreciate life to the fullest.** You do not take this moment for granted; therefore, you have no regrets.

   As you now know, there are a lot of benefits for you when you practice being present. Keep practicing and you will become a good curve ball hitter. You'll need to become good because, as you will see, life sometimes throws us more than one curve ball at a time.

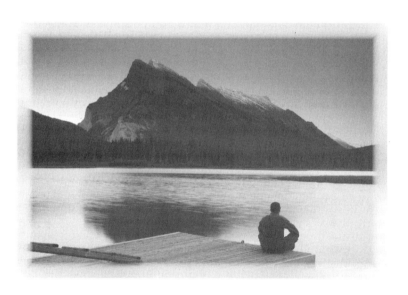

CHAPTER 5
IT'S TIME FOR THE F WORD (FAMILY)

It's Friday night, one day after my eye doctor's appointment, and I pick up the phone to call my seventy-year-old mother, who lives fifteen hundred miles away, in Boise, Idaho. Mom moved from Minnesota to Idaho after Dad died to be closer to my sister. My brother, Steve, lives in Nebraska. My nine-year-old daughter, Alissa, is the only relative I have in Minnesota.

During the phone conversation with my mother, I explain the situation to her and ask, "Mom, will you come and see me?""

She responds, "Roger, your sister, Linda, cannot go because she has to take care of Steve." Steve is my brother-in-law. He is severely disabled with cerebral palsy.

"I know Linda can't make the trip, Mom. I don't expect her to."

My mother continues, "Maybe it would be best if I came after the operation. You won't be able to move around much afterwards and that's when I will be the most helpful."

I laugh because I am obviously not getting through to her. "Mom, I might not be around after the operation."

She doesn't seem to understand my future plans do not extend past Thursday.

She continues, "Roger, I don't know if I can explain to the cab driver how to get from the airport to the hospital, and I don't know if I can get a flight by Tuesday. If I do come see you now, I will have to come back to take care of you after the operation."

After talking to my mom, I call my brother, Steve, and ask him, "Will you come and see me in the hospital before the operation?"

"I am not sure I can drive in the busy traffic surrounding the hospital, and I don't know if I will be able to even find the hospital," my brother replies.

I hang up on him.

He calls back and says, "I will be there."

I then call my sister, Linda, and ask her to influence my mother to come see me before the operation. Linda says, "I don't think Mom should go and see you until after the operation either."

I say, "If Mom doesn't come to see me before the operation and I die, I won't see her again. If she doesn't come and see me before the operation and I live, I don't want to see her again." The truth is I just want my mother to come running to comfort me like they do in the movies — but this isn't the movies.

After I am done talking on the phone, I feel like I have been kicked in the stomach. I have felt this pain before, way too many times. I feel this pain whenever I disappoint someone, or I am disappointed by someone. The emotional pain tonight is unbearable, and I began to cry. I realize now I have never felt loved. I also realize I have never loved myself. For the first time in my life, I admit to myself I don't love myself.

For as long as I can remember, I have always wanted to be perfect so I could get the love and respect I have craved. Now, as I face death, I realize I have no time to find someone to love me.

That leaves me — to love me.

I must trust, respect, forgive, and nurture myself in order to make the most out of the time I have left. For the first time in my life I feel loved, unconditionally, by me. I am crying and laughing at the same time. There is no time to look for love outside of myself. There is no time to be a victim.

I have to make the best use of my time and the best use of my time is to love myself. I forgive myself for everything I have done and said in the past that wasn't perfect. I forgive myself for possibly saying the wrong thing going forward. I know it's hard to believe I might say the wrong thing. Ha, I laugh at myself.

I have no choice now, but to be my self. I have no choice but to step back and let my real self take over.

For the first time in my life, my spirit is in control and I trust it. It is an odd feeling because, instead of trying to control everything and make it perfect, I am standing to the side and watching the real me.

In a perfect world, my family would be providing more (or some) emotional support. Oh yeah, I almost forgot for a second — in a perfect world I wouldn't have a baseball in my head, either.

Lesson Unlearned #5
What is the downside to living in the present?

Here is a summary of the benefits of living in the present from the last chapter.

1. You take responsibility for your actions.

2. There is less stress because you are concentrating on what you can control.

3. You have more energy.

4. You are aware, not only of your actions, but also of your thoughts.

5. You distinguish between your self-talk and your intuition.

6. You experience and appreciate life to the fullest.

The downside to living in the present is you expose your true self. When you live in the present, you are responsible for your actions. Your spirit is most precious, and it takes courage to expose your own vulnerability. You are never more vulnerable than when you live in the present because you cannot hide behind excuses about the past and wishes of the future.

You have to be there emotionally for yourself. You are the one who has to offer forgiveness to yourself when you need it. Nurture yourself when you need it. Praise yourself when you need it. This brings us to benefit number 7.

7. You love yourself.

Take a few minutes to review these seven benefits. Can you truly claim all of them for yourself? Especially number 7?

When you love yourself, you take responsibility for your own happiness and well-being. You respect yourself and naturally set boundaries to protect yourself physically, financially, and emotionally. When you have self respect, you will gain the respect of others.

You can start creating a happier life for yourself right now by loving yourself.

CHAPTER 6
THE INNOCENCE
OF A CHILD

Day Three

It's Saturday morning, two days after my eye doctor appointment. I am sitting in the living room of my apartment watching television with my nine-year-old daughter, Alissa. Alissa turns away from the television, looks at me, and confidently says, "There is good news and bad news about 1996, Dad."

"What's that?" I ask.

"The good news is I am going to turn ten this year, and the bad news is you have already turned forty!" she laughs.

I love the munchkin. She knows I am not crazy about turning forty. I laugh back and smile, as I shake my fist at her, while she laughs at me.

When she is done laughing, I say, "Alissa, come here, sit down by me, and let's shut off the television. I need to talk to you about something." When she comes over and sits by me, I hug her and then say, "I'm going to the hospital on Tuesday, and the doctors are going to remove something from behind my eye."

"What is it, Dad?" she asks.

"I really don't know what it is; it's just something that doesn't belong there."

I purposely avoid the brain tumor term. I want to be honest with her, but I don't want to scare her too much. I'm already scared enough for both of us. I know if I die or have a stroke, she will be hurt. I just hope to prepare her a little.

"We have to be positive, but we also have to be strong," I tell her. I go on to explain there is a chance I will end up like her uncle who has cerebral palsy and is in a wheelchair.

"I could die, but then again, I could get hit by a car tomorrow and die. We both have to be strong and positive at the same time. Are you all right?" I ask.

"Yes, Dad, I'll pray for you."

"I love you, Alissa."

"I love you, too, Dad."

I spend the rest of the day looking at Alissa and engraving a picture of her deep into my mind. Nothing else seems to matter except for engraving a deep picture of Alissa into my mind and my conversations with God, which are continuous.

Later, at night I lie down in my bed to go to sleep. I began to talk to God for the one hundredth time today. I have this feeling like I am going to the principal's office on Thursday. Only, this principal (God) not only knows everything I have ever done, but also knows every thought I have ever had.

All I can do is hope God is a merciful God. I know it's hard to believe, but I certainly haven't lived my life like a saint and I have had my share of juicy thoughts.

I lie still and begin praying, "God, I know you are there, and I am never going to question that. I trust your will. I'm not going to pray for myself, but what about Alissa? She has been through so much."

Then I realize praying for Alissa is just another way of praying for myself. "God, I know you are there, and I am not going to pray for an outcome. You know I want to live, but whatever your will is, I accept it."

Without mentioning it in my prayer, I cannot help but think the worst outcome, and the most likely outcome, would be somewhere in between life and death. I certainly do not want to suffer a stroke or some kind of serious brain damage. "Two things are for sure, God, I'm going to approach this with a sense of humor, and I put my faith in your will. Thank you, God, for everything."

I realize at this moment, I am God's child, nothing more, nothing less.

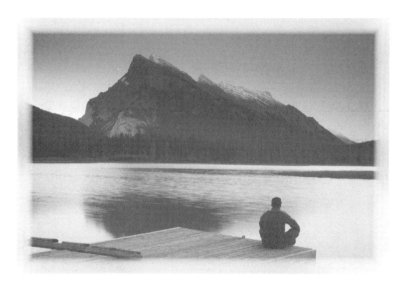

Lesson Unlearned #6
Love Your Inner Child as if
He or She Were Your Own

It's easy to love a child because children are so innocent and playful. Each one of us has a child inside of us. The inner child is the foundation of who we really are. Our inner child, soul, spirit, and higher self are all one in the same. For my purposes here, I will call the part of the subconscious mind that is not affected by outside stimulus the spirit. Unlike the ego, the spirit is innate. The ego is affected by outside stimulus. The ego tries to avoid negative outside stimulus and it desires more positive stimulus.

On the other hand, the spirit is not affected by outside stimulus. The spirit affects the outside world through inspiration, intuition, and energy. If you want to reap the benefits of genius from your soul, spirit, and higher self, you must love your inner child.

When you nurture and love your inner child, you trust your spirit, and encourage your spirit to show its true self. When your spirit shines through you, you become the most authentic you who you can be.

This doesn't mean you should say or do everything your inner child wants, but you have to acknowledge it. Do not apologize for being yourself. It's the beginning of suppressing your spirit. If you suppress your inner child, you are suppressing your spirit and your true self. You are denying who you really are. This is what I did for the first forty years of my life. I thought that by changing myself, I would get the love and acceptance I had dreamed of. No one noticed. All suppressing my spirit did was make me angry because no one noticed. Also, by trying to change my personality, I became afraid to trust my real personality.

Close your eyes and imagine a time when you were young and needed love but did not receive it from anyone. Picture yourself at that time and visualize what you looked like then. Feel the pain you felt then.

Now imagine yourself as you are today. Imagine walking up to the child who is in emotional pain. Imagine giving your young self the unconditional love you desired, needed, and deserved.

Hug the child in you who made a mistake. Give yourself a smile and a high five for all of the incredible things you have done. Whatever love was missing in the child's life, imagine yourself today stepping back in time and giving the child that love.

When you feel emotional pain, nurture yourself as you would nurture your child. Be your own parent and your own best friend. Instead of overeating or indulging in alcohol and drugs, hug yourself.

Look in a mirror and tell yourself you love you. Hold yourself and love yourself unconditionally until the pain goes away. Does this seem silly? Then laugh at yourself. Laughing is a good thing. It means you are present.

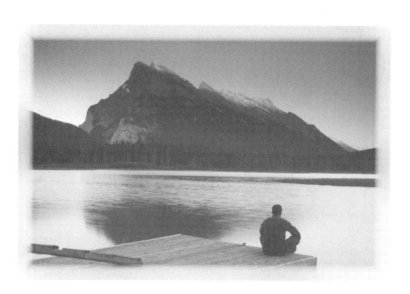

CHAPTER 7
CLOSE ONLY COUNTS IN HORSESHOES AND EMBOLIZATION
Day Six

On Thursday I went to the eye doctor. Now it is the following Tuesday morning, and I have just been admitted into the hospital. I am lying on a table wearing one of those funky hospital robes. Young female nurses are coming in and out of the room. A nurse about my age (forty) comes in the room after being briefed by one of the younger nurses. She has an in-charge serious look. She tells me the surgeon has changed the plan slightly, and I will have both an angiogram and an embolization today. This way, I will have a day of rest before the surgery on Thursday.

She says, "Somebody will return and began prepping you for the angiogram." She adds, "Somebody will be in shortly to shave your groin."

"What?" I blurt out. "What does shaving my groin have to do with brain surgery?" I ask, knowing it is a leading question.

"You know what they say about where men's brains are," she responds.

That was a good shot; I laugh, but before I finish laughing, my spirit retaliates back. "This sounds like the beginning of my sexual harassment suit."

She looks more than a little rattled by my quick comeback, not realizing at first I am just having fun. Then she smiles, laughs, and says, "You set me up."

I tell her I appreciate her sense of humor and she tells me she appreciates mine. *I probably won't be alive after Thursday, and she's afraid I am going to sue her. Now that's FUNNY!*

After the nurses finish prepping me, an attendant pushes me into the radiation area. All I know about an angiogram is they are going to shoot a dye in my veins so they can take pictures. An embolization, I have learned, is a process that cuts off the blood supply to the tumor, so it is easier for the surgeon to operate.

All I am doing is lying still on the table while the doctor and technician do their thing. At first it seems simple, but now the male technician keeps telling me to stay still. I think I am lying still, but he keeps telling me I'm not. I'm trying to relax. All I have to do is lie still, and I can't even do that right. Finally, I get through it.

After they are done, a nurse comes in the room and asks me if anybody is waiting for me. I tell her yes, and the nurse says she will go and tell her she can come in now. My new-found friend drove me to the hospital, and she said she would wait around until the procedure was done. In a few minutes, the nurse comes back and tells me there isn't anybody waiting for me, but she left a message with the desk clerk to tell her to come in if she comes back.

"She must have left you for somebody else," the technician says to me.

I wish he wouldn't give me a bad time right now.

"Yeah, she must have took off and left you," he says, as if he thinks he's funny.

I really wish he would quit this. I know he's just kidding, but I'm not in the greatest mood after he just scolded me for not being able to lie still. He doesn't know it, but he could be right. She's just a friend and didn't promise to wait.

"It doesn't look like she's coming back," he says for the third time.

That's it. He's had his fun, now it's my turn.

"Could you come here for a minute?" I ask this because I'm strapped down, I can't move, and I can't see his face clearly. He comes over so I can see him. He's a pretty big guy, over six feet, and in his early thirties. In a firm voice with a smile on my face, I ask,

"Have you ever been beat up by a guy with a brain tumor before?"

He looks at me with a straight face and says, "No, not many guys have ever done that."

I grin as he goes back and finishes his work, nice and quietly, which is all I wanted in the first place. We both know if I was ten years younger and had a baseball bat, he would still beat me up, but we also both know he is in a no-win situation.

Whenever I blurt something out without thinking, I feel guilty because so many times in my life I have been told to think before I speak. I worry about saying the wrong thing. This time is different, though. The guilt goes away immediately because I have no time for guilt. The guilt thought passes through my mind because I don't dwell on it, identify with it, or attach to it. It's a waste of time and time is everything. I have to spend my time concentrating on what's going on.

I could have just asked the male radiological technician to be quiet, but that wouldn't have been me. *Worst case scenario, everything goes well, and he tracks me down and kicks my butt.* I laugh to myself, That's like the best case scenario, right now. I continue laughing to myself.

I have to wait and see what I have to work with on Thursday. That's when my part starts. Until then, I just have to keep my sense of humor. That's my promise to myself and to God. I am going to keep my sense of humor, and I am going to do the best I can, after the operation, with the cards I am dealt. If I have to spend the rest of my life learning how to walk and talk, that's what I am going to do. That is my promise.

After they push me to my room, the surgeon comes in and tells me they were able to cut off 90 percent of the blood supply to the tumor. He appears very pleased with the results of the embolization.

Thursday is still the make-or-break day.

Oh, I almost forgot to tell you, my new-found nurse friend showed up shortly after I got to my room. At about seven o'clock at night my mother and my brother came into my room. I was so glad to see them.

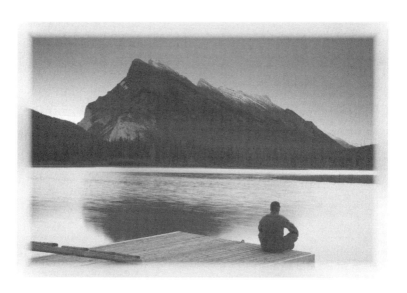

Lesson Unlearned #7
Forgive Yourself

Think back to some of the worst things you have ever done in your life. What did you learn from those mistakes that will help you move forward?

Ask yourself, honestly, if it was your ego that caused you to do something bad or your spirit? If you are truly honest, you will see it was most likely your ego. If it was your ego, you must learn to quit letting your ego control and wreck your life.

If it truly was your spirit that caused the mistake, you must learn from your mistake, forgive yourself, and move forward. Don't apologize for your spirit, or you will repress it. There is another answer. Here is the secret to positive change.

You do not have to change your personality, nor can you.

You can change your outlook on life.

If you truly and sincerely appreciate everything about this moment, your outlook on life will be so good, your spirit will soar, and you will not hurt anyone, nor will anyone be able to hurt you.

The authenticity that results from the combination of appreciating everything right now and being your true self is what makes living in the present so special.

Concentrate on having a positive and happy outlook on life, and you will be surprised how pleasant and likeable your personality becomes. There will be no reason to feel guilt or shame. If you do have negative feelings, let them go, concentrate on being appreciative and having a happy outlook on life. If your true self makes a mistake, forgive yourself, put the mistake in perspective, learn from it, laugh at it, and keep going.

Don't use blaming yourself and others as an excuse to hold you back. Forgive yourself to move forward and live the life you were born to live.

Now let's move forward with day seven of my journey.

CHAPTER 8
HAPPY ST. VALENTINE'S DAY
Day Seven

It's Wednesday, February 14, 1996, six days after my eye doctor appointment and one day before my surgery. The surgeon has planned this as a rest day, and my mother, brother, and I have planned a little Valentine's Day party for my daughter, Alissa. The nurses are letting us hold the party in one of the waiting rooms. At the end of the party, I ask Alissa to come with me to my room. I feel a lot of anxiety, and I wonder if this is the last time I will ever see her. She is very calm and she doesn't understand the significance.

After the party, Alissa and I are left alone in my room for a few minutes. I try to keep it short. "I love you, Alissa."

"I love you, too, Dad."

"Alissa, no matter what happens, or what anybody says, always remember there is a God and always pray."

"OK, Dad," she says.

"I love you, honey," I say, as we start to walk out of the room.

"I love you, too, Dad." We say goodnight to each other as she leaves the hospital.

Based on the advice of my new-found nurse friend, my brother and I discuss the possible outcomes of the surgery, while my nurse friend takes my mother for a walk.

"We have to discuss the possibility I might be brain dead after the surgery," I tell my brother.

"What do you want me to do?" my brother, Steve, asks.

"I'm not a quitter, and I don't plan on quitting now, but if there's absolutely no chance, I don't want Alissa to have to tell people her dad is lying in a room somewhere, but he doesn't know who he is, or who she is.

"My job starts tomorrow after the surgery. I have to see what I have to work with. It's up to me to do the best I can with the cards I'm dealt. It all depends on God's will through the skill of the surgeon's hands what those cards are going to be."

As I lie in the hospital bed, my sister, Linda, calls to wish me good luck. I tell her I am approaching this with a positive attitude and a sense of humor. "I'm looking forward to waking up sometime tomorrow, and I am going to hit the ground running," I tell her.

"Or maybe open up one eye," she says.

As I lie in the hospital the night before the surgery, I have never felt so peaceful. It is as though I have spent my entire life trying to control something or somebody, or I felt that somebody was trying to control me. Now

I feel free from control and attachment. All I want to do is live.

Before last week, I thought I was the center of the universe, yet I did not value my time on earth. Now I realize how insignificant my life is in comparison to the universe and in comparison to how long the earth has been in existence. But I also realize how valuable my life and my time on earth are.

For some reason, this new attitude makes me feel amazingly calm while at the same time making me unbelievably aware of what is going on inside of me and around me.

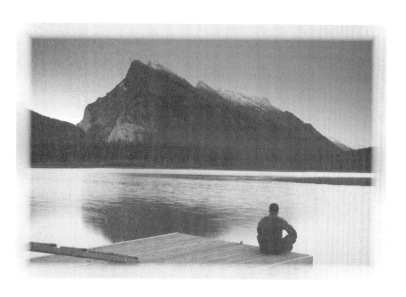

Lesson Unlearned #8
Creating Happiness

Manifestation is based on the law of cause and effect, which means if you think a certain way, a predictable outcome is inevitable. Based on this principle, the ultimate example of the Law of Cause and Effect is simply this:

When you sincerely appreciate the fact that you are alive right now, it is impossible not to be happy right now.

Happiness is inevitable if you appreciate everything about your life right now, this very moment. You must not take life for granted. You could have died earlier, or you may not have been born at all. Instead of trying to be happy, create an atmosphere where happiness is inevitable. Appreciating every aspect of your life will create such an atmosphere.

This may sound too simple because it is. The ego will try to trick you into believing there is some complicated formula you must find to be happy. The ego will try to tell you that you need more — more of this, more of that, if you only had what someone else has. Blah, blah, blah.

Yet, true happiness comes from the relationships you enjoy with yourself, with family, with co-workers, with old friends, with new friends, with nature, with life itself, and with God, if you're so inclined. Happiness doesn't come from having more, from being liked, or from wishing time away. Give yourself the gift of happiness by appreciating your life today.

CHAPTER 9
GAME DAY
(Boys and girls, please don't try this at home)
Day Eight

It's 6:30, Thursday morning, one week after my eye doctor appointment. The nurse wakes me up, and puts strange long white nylon socks on me. The attendant comes in the room with a wheelchair. I get in the chair and the attendant wheels me into the pre-op room. The surgical nurse asks me to sign a consent form for the operation. She comes back a few minutes later, and asks me to sign another consent form. This form is to give consent to cut my hair.

"I signed a consent form that says you can cut into my head. I guess it's OK to cut my hair. Can you keep my hair for me after its cut?" I ask, chuckling.

"We could do that, but we never have before. Why?" she asks with a perplexed look.

"When my friends give me a bad time for losing my hair, I can hold up a plastic bag with the hair in it and say, 'I've still got it right here,'" I respond.

The nurse shakes her head, smiling as she turns and leaves.

My mother and brother come into the pre-op room. The surgeon also comes in to say hi, but only briefly because he has to get ready. My brother comments that the surgeon looks like he has a fresh haircut and a new suit. "He looks like he's having a good day," my brother says.

I chuckle to myself; professional athletes have their good days and their bad days, I hope the surgeon is on his game today.

The attendant comes in the room, and I tell my mom and my brother I love them and give them the thumbs up. As I am wheeled into the operating room, I began to pray.

"God, I love you. God, thank you for letting me live. You have listened to my prayers. It's time for me to listen to you. I am prepared to meet you."

I have never felt such peace. The anesthesiologist starts to put an I. V. in my arm.

This would be a great experience — if it just wasn't real.

Lesson Unlearned #9
Peace

Death is reality. No amount of positive thinking is going to keep you alive forever, but perspective will give you peace. Peace comes from trusting your own spirit and accepting God's will.

Getting mad at God because life isn't perfect is like getting a free, all-inclusive vacation to Hawaii from an anonymous donor, then calling up the anonymous donor and yelling at him or her because you are sunburned.

You cannot change death, but you can change your life and become an inspiration.

Directions to a Peaceful Life

Appreciate life itself.
Nurture and develop your inner child so it can find its
purposeful path.
Trust your spirit and follow your purposeful path.
At times, the path will be paved with gold.
At times, the path will be nearly impossible to follow.
Smile, laugh, trust your spirit, and accept God's will.
Continue to follow your path.
When you get to the graveyard, you went too far.

We all get to the graveyard someday, but what can we do to create a wonderful journey before then? We can give ourselves permission to trust our spirit, and to appreciate life. We make our journey as good as possible when we do.

CHAPTER 10
A WHOLE NEW BALL GAME

As I lie on the operating table, the anesthesiologist finishes inserting the I.V. in my arm. The next thing I know I am transported to a new place.

I am sitting on a large flat rock on the edge of a spectacular mountain lake. The lake is more beautiful than any lake I have ever seen, or ever imagined. The water is crystal clear and as smooth as glass on this perfectly calm day. The temperature is just right. The sun shines brightly, and there are no clouds in the magnificent blue sky.

EVERYTHING IS PERFECT!

Mountains surround the lake and rise far up into the sky. I sit quietly and calmly on the rock with shorts and no shirt as my bare feet dangle in the water. My eyes and ears are glued to the sky. My sight is clearer than ever, my hearing is sharper than ever, and I feel more energy than ever. The energy brings a special peace.

God is speaking to me as sure as the sun is shining. Later, I will not be able to recall what he said, but he is talking and I am listening. I feel completely accepted by God's unconditional love. I am at peace and excited at the same time. I am mesmerized by God's omniscient (all knowing) presence as I listen in awe. I smile uncontrollably.

I close my eyes and I inhale as the palms of my hands come together and my arms reach above my head and then separate as I pull my arms down and feel my body thrust upward. I swim upwards, but there is no water. There is only darkness and a small bright light. I am swimming through the night air towards the bright light. I smile and feel the energy rush through me. I take another stroke as my body surges forward. The light glimmers above. The light is brighter and closer as I inhale while my arms perform another stroke upward. I exhale and open my eyes.

Yes!

There are two hospital lights hanging above me and I can see the lights as clearly as I could see the blue sky a moment ago. I lie still in the hospital bed after taking my first new breath. This is the most significant breath in my life.

It is a breath I did not expect to experience. I am not concerned with what I look like, how much money I make, who likes me, or even how I feel. Those thoughts don't cross my mind. No thoughts cross my mind. I am breathing. *I am alive.*

I can see clearly out of my right eye. For the first time in weeks, there is no fog in front of my right eye when I first wake up.

WHAM. *Oh my God, forget those fantastic feelings. The top of my head just exploded. I feel the most intense pain of my life. I think I'm screaming, but I don't know if I am physically capable of screaming. I am definitely screaming on the inside with all of my might.*

This is perhaps a small taste of how a newborn baby feels. I am so excited and joyful to be alive. I am full of wonder about this world, a world I didn't expect to see. I want to experience it with all of my energy and savor it for as long as I can. At the same time, the pain is indescribably excruciating. It hurts so much, yet I am incredibly thankful I am able to feel the pain. Like a newborn baby, I cannot talk or communicate the unbelievable combination of pain and joy.

I am thankful I am able to breathe. I am thankful to be able to see. I am thankful I am passing out now.

Even though I just passed out from the intense pain, I am so thankful. Thank you, God, thank you.

***Take a deep breath
and imagine it is your very first breath.***

Live every day as if it were your first day,
with the zest and enthusiasm of a child.
Don't stop and smell the roses;
Instead, run directly to the roses.

All of my needs are met. If I die right now, I have exceeded my expectations. I have had one more breath than I expected.

I wake up for the second time. I cannot see out of my right eye; it's swollen shut. I don't care because I know the fog is gone.

I have no desires, no needs, no judgments, and no thoughts. I have no mind. All I have is energy, a peaceful, yet powerful energy. I appreciate everything. I take nothing for granted. I have never had less, and I have never been happier.

Now it's test time. First, I wiggle the toes on my left foot. Then I wiggle the toes on my right foot. Now, I wiggle the fingers on my left hand. Lastly, I wiggle the fingers on my right hand.

I am so excited and so happy. The excitement and overwhelming joy only lasts for a minute, though, because the excruciating pain returns or my thoughts remind me the pain was there all of the time. I pass out again.

The third time I wake up, I see a nurse above me. She tells me the tumor was benign, not cancerous. *Benign is arguably the best word in the whole English language.* The nurse then tells me the surgeon was able to remove 100 percent of the tumor. *That's a good thing.* Even though I know the surgeon used the most sophisticated technology, I would swear somebody took an ice pick to my head. I keep laughing inside because I know a world-record headache is a small price to pay for life.

The nurse tells me the surgery lasted nine hours. *Nine hours, I could have sworn I took a twenty-minute nap.* The nurse asks me to rate my headache on a scale of one to ten; ten being the worst.

"*An eight,*" I respond, comparing it to the excruciating pain I experienced earlier when I woke up the first time.

She asks me if I would like more morphine.

I smile, "If you're selling, I am buying."

I fall asleep again and have the same dream of the spectacular mountain lake.

Later, a different nurse wakes me up to do some tests. She tells me to touch my nose and wiggle my feet. I am very groggy and can barely do the tests, but I do my best. She asks me where I am.

"I was on the most beautiful mountain lake until you interrupted me and brought me back to this hospital," I answer.

I spend my waking moments in intensive care thanking God. I thank God I am alive and for my ability to move all of my body parts. I pray for all of the people I know who have died. I pray for all people who are paralyzed. I pray with all of my heart.

Lesson Unlearned #10
Happiness 101

Why was I so happy right after my operation?

The obvious answer is really good *medication*. That is not completely accurate, though, because even with plenty of good medication I was still in great pain. There are other reasons:

1. I was living in the present.

2. I appreciated everything.

3. It was a secret.

You must be present to pass Happiness 101. Never, ever before in my life had I experienced the deep happiness and joy I experienced when I first woke up from my surgery. Never had I concentrated so intensely on the Now. I had no expectations. Every breath was extra. I took nothing for granted. Everything was special — even the pain.

I was too busy concentrating on breathing and seeing to think about the past and the future. I had no mind to create labels, judgments, and limitations to stop the flow of energy.

How can this help those of us who have to deal with the pressures of society and the day-to-day struggle to meet expectations, deadlines, and keep our heads above water while the waves are crashing up against us from different directions?

We must first realize today's society is predominantly ruled by egos. Next, we must realize the ego world is not reality. Our minds are not reality. Being present is reality, but you do not have to tell anyone you care more about breathing, seeing, hearing, smelling, tasting, and touching than you do about impressing someone. Living in the present is the first reason I was so happy.

The second reason I was so happy is because I appreciated everything. Think of a time when you were the most appreciative in your life. What did it feel like? Close your eyes and visualize what it was like when you were so appreciative. Practice meditating on this scene so you can recreate the appreciative feeling whenever you want. You have had this feeling before. You can recreate it through visualization. An attitude of abundance is the opposite of an attitude of fear. When you have an attitude of fear, your self-talk says things back to you like, "What if this bad thing happens, or what if that happens?" When you have an attitude of abundance, your self-talk says things back to you like, "I am so happy. Thank you."

The third reason I was so happy is because it was a secret. Living in the present and appreciating everything creates positive energy. When you keep your happiness a secret, the positive energy does not dissipate or disperse. Instead the positive energy stays concentrated within you and multiplies. You will radiate and the positive energy will seep out of you, as it should.

Of course, unfortunately, you may have experienced the opposite. If you vent negative energy it goes away, at least temporarily, until you create more negative energy. But if you withhold the negative energy it just gets worse until you feel like you are going to explode.

Now, you know how to create positive energy by living in the present and appreciating everything. You also know how to store the positive energy by keeping your happiness a secret. Your body will ooze positive energy and happiness for all of those around you to see and sense.

Of course, this happened to me without me knowing what was happening. I just knew I was happy and that I couldn't explain it, so why try. Living your life with the proper perspective and keeping it a secret has its advantages.

1. It keeps your ego in check. By not telling anyone why you are so happy, you don't put yourself above anyone.

2. Other egos will not be able to attack you and put you down. Once you realize the difference between your own spirit and your ego, you will start to notice the difference between other people's spirits and their egos. The ego is always trying to better the spirit and put it down. Now you know how you can protect your spirit with your own unconditional love.

3. No one will believe you when you tell them why you are so happy anyway because all you are doing is appreciating the little things in life.

That Lucky Feeling

Deep gratitude for life itself leads to an attitude of abundance.
An attitude of abundance creates a lucky feeling.
This lucky feeling is positive energy.
When you are thankful for the lucky feeling, the positive energy multiplies.

One of the keys to getting what you desire is not to need anything. When you have a feeling of abundance, your desires come freely to you because there is no resistance. If you practice this appreciative visualization exercise, you will enjoy this feeling of abundance. Go to your place of appreciation often (mine is sitting on the rock by the beautiful mountain lake) and create an attitude of abundance. Practice nurturing your spirit, creating an attitude of abundance and keeping it a secret. Soon you will be passing Happiness 101 with an uncontrollable smile.

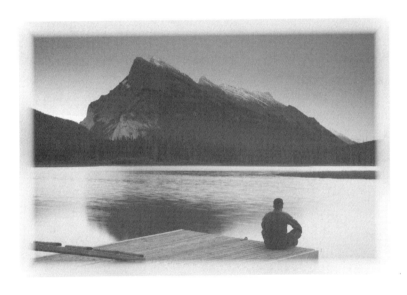

CHAPTER 11
BULGING BICEPS, ROCK HARD ABS, AND BRAINS OF STEEL

Day Ten

It's Saturday morning, nine days after my eye doctor appointment and two days after my operation. I spent most of Friday listening to God talk to me while I sat beside the beautiful mountain lake I described earlier. I spent the rest of Friday screaming in pain. Now on Saturday morning, an attendant is moving me from the intensive care unit to another floor. The pain is excruciating as the attendant apologizes for going over bumps in the hallway. I am in so much pain, it doesn't make any difference whether or not we are going over any bumps. I feel like the attendant could push me off a cliff, and the pain wouldn't be any worse.

I'm whining. I catch myself and snap back to reality. The pain is only a seven on a one-to-ten scale. I remind myself I am alive and I can move all of my body parts.

I spend all day Saturday trying not to move because any movement causes my headache to become more intense. I cannot even roll over without grabbing the railing on the side of the bed and moving real slow. Even with all of the pain, I am so happy and free.

Somehow, something has opened a door
and released a hidden part of me.
It is as though my physical self
and my true self are two separate entities.
The tremendous physical pain keeps me from moving,
but it is overshadowed
by the excitement of my spirit
dancing and savoring every glorious moment.

It has been two days since I woke up from my surgery and my daughter, Alissa, is coming to visit me today for the first time since the surgery. I am excited. I am also nervous because I have a bandage covering half of my head. I must look like a wounded soldier in a war movie.

Alissa comes in the room and seems to be OK with everything because she was told what to expect. After a short visit, my mother, brother, and Alissa go to lunch while I take a nap. When they come back, I wake up, and my right eye pops open. I'm happy because Alissa gets to see me with both of my eyes open, and I get to see her with both of my eyes.

It's later in the evening now and all of my visitors are gone. I try to walk with the nurse's help. I can only take three very small steps because the pain is too intense to go any further. I am bothered because a sixty-year-old patient walks by my room, stops, looks at me, and continues walking. I'm only forty years old, and I can barely stand up. The nurses say I'm doing well though; that's nice. I can tell the nurses are a little bit taken aback by my excitement and enthusiasm. One of the nurses tells me she has never seen a patient so ecstatic about having his head split open.

Now it's noon on Sunday, three days after my operation, and my mother and brother leave to go back to their homes. I needed and appreciated their company before and after the surgery. I am so thankful everything turned out so well, but I still have to battle this nasty headache and a couple of other issues: the catheter and constipation. How embarrassing!

I'm just happy my head is still on.

Now it's midnight, and two nurses later. The night nurse is nice. She jokes around and then has me do a bunch of silly tests and exercises. She tells me to remember three words: dog, ball, and rosebud. She has me touch my nose with my eyes closed and move my legs and arms. As she's leaving the room, I tell her I think she forgot something. She asks what, and I say, "dog, ball, and rosebud."

She laughs and tells me about a time when a patient could only remember two of the three words, but she couldn't remember the third word either.

It's Monday morning, four days after my operation and the clinical nurse specialist comes to see me. She is very attractive. She tells me I am doing great, and I have a positive attitude. I appreciate her good feedback. She takes the bandage off my head. After she leaves, I manage to make my way to the bathroom mirror, half walking and half crawling.

I look in the mirror. So much for my positive attitude, I look like an outer-space alien in a science fiction movie. The front half of my head is shaved and my right eye looks like a professional heavyweight boxer punched me (more than once). There are stitches running above my left ear, following my hair line, all the way to my right ear. I think someone told me there were fifty-eight stitches.

Some women have told me I have a nice full head of brown hair to go with my big brown eyes. Now half of my hair is completely gone with a big bloody scar across the front of my head. I laugh at myself as I look in the mirror because I realize I might have had big brown eyes because the tumor was making them bulge.

Maybe I'll tell women it's a new hair style. It's called a Lifesaver Haircut. It's ugly, it costs more than you can believe, and it hurts more than you can imagine, but it's a lifesaver. I wonder if my hair will ever come back. Then I start laughing, as I look down and see a plastic bag by the side of my bed with my hair in it. After teasing myself for losing my perspective, I crawl back to my nice safe bed. I am sure it is my imagination, but I swear I can feel my brain sloshing around inside of my head because it is no longer attached. I continue laughing at myself until I fall asleep.

Don't judge a book by its cover.
Unless of course,
there is nothing inside of the book.

By the way, that line is referring to my head, not this book!

It's much later now, 1:00 a.m. Tuesday morning, five days after my operation. The night nurse just finished her usual routine and told me I need more rest. I agree with her, and tell her I haven't slept more than an hour or two at a time since the surgery.

She responds, "Patients are like babies, they have to learn how to sleep through the night."

At 1:30 a.m., I lie restless in my hospital bed. I still can't sleep. Then much to my surprise, the door opens and two female friends sneak into the room.

One of them is my new-found nurse friend who took me to the hospital. It's obvious they've been out having a good time and decided to stop by and give me a bad time. I think it makes all three of us feel young, like we're breaking the rules. One of them changes the board on the wall, which lists my required daily activities. She erases walking as the activity, and writes, "push-ups, sit-ups, and lifting weights." The other one says, "He doesn't have to exercise. He doesn't need rock hard abs, or bulging biceps, he's got **Brains of Steel**; that's all he needs." They leave, and I laugh myself to sleep.

I spend Tuesday, Wednesday, and Thursday walking up and down the hallway looking for the sixty-year-old man who walked by my room the other day, so I can ask him if he wants to race.

One of the nurses asks me to rate my headache again. I tell her, "It's only a two, but believe me, I know what a ten feels like."

She says, "Men. You don't know what pain is until you've delivered a baby."

I laugh, "You are right. I don't know what it's like to have a baby, but I feel like the doctor took a baby out of my head!"

I spend evenings in the hospital talking to visitors, relatives, and friends on the phone. My room is full of flowers, plants, and balloons. The nurses are giving me a bad time for having too many visitors, and being on the phone too much. It's great!

Self discipline is fine, but not self deprivation.
There is enough real pain in life;
Creating artificial pain is for amateurs.

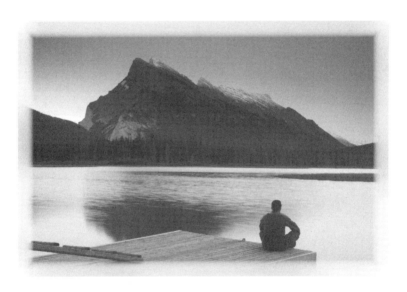

Lesson Unlearned #11
Don't Forget to Laugh!

As soon as I woke up from my operation, my sense of humor was heightened for two reasons: I had a big picture perspective and something I call the brilliance of resilience.

Reality of death is a gift because it puts life in proper perspective and helps us laugh. Here is the big picture perspective:

> *Life is a gift.*
> *Appreciate everything good about life,*
> *no matter how small it is,*
> *because life is a gift and it does end.*
> *Do not dwell on anything bad in life,*
> *no matter how big it is,*
> *because life is a gift and it does end.*

After my operation, I accepted myself because of my dream about God accepting me, and I had a big picture perspective.

In addition to a big picture perspective, I also had something I call the brilliance of resilience. The brilliance of resilience means you can do anything if you have to do it. The brilliance of resilience is raw determination. No one can make you have a raw determination mind-set but yourself.

When I was in college, I got straight As because I believed my back was to the wall and I was determined. I was laid off, I had a baby daughter, and I believed I was going to have a difficult time finding a first job out of college because I was thirty-four. Also, because it had been eight years since I got out of the Air Force, I only had two years of the GI bill left when I started college. My caseworker at the unemployment office told me I might be able to get my last two years of books and tuition paid, if the displaced worker program was still in place, and if my grades were good. I couldn't control whether or not the government funding would still be in place, so I concentrated on what I could control — my grades.

The question is what is your brain tumor? What would it take for you to promise your self and/or God that you will be happy?

The Brilliance of Resilience

Adversity is directly related to living in the present.
Adversity forces you to focus all of your
energy on what you can control.
You concentrate on little steps and

you take one day at a time.
What if you had to be happy and there
was no time for anything else?
What if you focused all of your energy
on being happy right now?
What if you said the following two sentences?
"Someday, I will be happy, and I'll be
darned if today isn't some day."
"I promise myself and God I will be happy today."
What then?

If you combine the following five principles, it's difficult not to be happy:

1. Develop an attitude of abundance.

2. Keep a big picture perspective.

3. Promise God you will be happy. Do everything in your power to keep your promise.

4. Take little steps. Live in the present and concentrate fully on those little steps.

5. Don't forget to laugh.

Life is a journey; enjoy the trip.
Don't bring any baggage, but never,
ever forget your sense of humor.

Don't be afraid to love because,
without it, you cannot really live.
Don't be afraid to feel pain because,
without it, you cannot grow.
There will be times when you need to be strong.
Remember how tough you can be
and always remember that the ultimate strength
comes from your trust in God's will.

I have mentioned laughter often. I will continue to do so. Why? Raw determination and laughter are a powerful combination. Laughter is a great physical and mental exercise. Laughter is directly related to your outlook on life. If you have a positive outlook on life, your smile and laugh will show it. Laughter is a sign of being present and it is contagious. So don't forget to laugh.

CHAPTER 12
JUST YOUR BASIC, ROUTINE FRONTO-TEMPORAL CRANIOTOMY

Surprisingly, my brain tumor operation turned out to be the greatest experience of my life, with the exception of the birth of my daughter. I am fortunate I suffered no serious complications during or after the surgery. Some people have a stroke or severe short-term memory loss. One man told me he had a friend who lost his personality. I was so sad when I heard this because ironically, I feel like I found my personality, which had been lost for most of my life before the surgery.

Many things had to come together for the surgery to be successful. The eye doctor had to make the proper diagnosis and respond in a timely manner. It's not easy to tell somebody they might have a brain tumor, especially somebody as open-minded as me (Not!).

I used to have an open mind, but the surgeon took the tumor out and closed it back up. (Just a little inside joke.)

My eye doctor put up with the best denial tactics I could throw at him. He not only acted as a professional, he acted as a good Samaritan and a friend. He went above and beyond the call of duty by following up at night, and throughout my hospital stay and recovery.

At the very least, the eye doctor saved me from having a grand mal seizure, and I most likely would have died if the tumor had ruptured before the doctors discovered it.

I am fortunate to live in a day and age where we have the technology to perform such a complicated surgery. If I had lived in a prior generation, I would have died, and nobody would have even known what caused it.

I am very, very fortunate to have such a talented and skillful surgeon. I cannot imagine the intelligence, knowledge, and the concentration he must have to be able to do such detailed work for nine hours. Since the tumor was so large, there was no room for error, and he was able to get it all out. The surgeon's skill not only saved my life, but also saved my quality of life. Even the slightest slip can cause a permanent deficit such as loss of eye sight, memory loss, numbness, or loss of feeling in parts of the body, not to mention the possibility of being paralyzed for the rest of my life.

The surgeon was always straightforward with me, and he never made me feel inadequate because I didn't know what an embolization or a meningioma was. A meningioma is a tumor arising from the coverings of the brain rather than the brain itself. Usually, meningiomas are benign. The surgeon was nice, and he even put up with my sense of humor, knowing I was scared to death.

Most importantly, I am thankful for God's will. I believe if it wasn't for God's will, none of the above would have taken place. God gave me a second chance at life, a second chance to be a happy positive human being. He gave me a second chance to live in the present and appreciate every day.

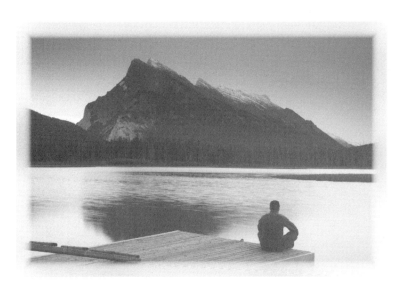

Lesson Unlearned #12
How can you learn to be present without having a traumatic experience?

The key to living in the present is to become aware of your actions and your thoughts. When you are present, you enter a heightened state of awareness because you are engrossed in activity. The following exercises are designed to help you increase your awareness and help you remember the times when you were present.

Exercise #1
Breathing is a physical activity. Sit quietly in your favorite chair when no one else is around. Close your eyes and breathe. Don't move at all, just sit still and breathe smoothly, continuously, and comfortably: In and out. Notice your thoughts as you concentrate on your breathing. Let the thoughts go and keep concentrating on your breathing.

If your mind wanders to something else, bring it back and concentrate on your breathing. Practice this for five minutes a day, working up to fifteen minutes a day. Once you get to fifteen minutes a session, start practicing the exercise twice a day. Notice you get better at concentrating on your breathing, and over time, there will be fewer thoughts crossing your mind. Also, your mind won't wander as much. If you fall asleep, don't worry about it. Next time keep concentrating on experiencing your breathing. Each time you are done, open your eyes, look around, and spend a minute to be thankful for everything and tell yourself you love yourself.

Exercise #2:
Practice an attitude of abundance. Once you are comfortable with exercise number one, replace it with a meditation on thankfulness. As you meditate, concentrate on being thankful for each breath. Breathe in and out, smoothly concentrating on being thankful for each breath. When you are done, you will have a feeling of thankfulness. As you continue to practice this exercise, you will notice an attitude of thankfulness throughout your day.

Exercise #3:
This exercise is similar to the earlier exercise of learning how to be present, but will help you reach a new level of staying in the present.

To perform this exercise, stand up with a clock in sight. Breathe, just as you were when you were sitting down, nice and smoothly. Look around and experience your eyes moving around as you look around the room. Experience what your eyes see. Listen and experience what you hear. Smell and experience what you smell. Lick your lips and experience what you taste. Move your hands and fingers around, experience your hands moving around. Now do all six activities at the same time: breathe, look, listen, smell, taste, and touch. Do not define, label, or judge what you see, hear, smell, taste, or feel. Do this for one minute. Progressively work your way up to five minutes. When you are done with this exercise, notice your senses are heightened because the flow of energy is not disrupted by thought.

Also notice what thoughts brought you out of the present. These thoughts mean your ego is trying to tell you that either your past or future is more important than reality, which, of course, is not true. After you have worked your way up to five minutes, add walking to the mix. Now move your hands and fingers as you walk and pay attention to all of your senses at the same time. Start with one minute and work your way up to five minutes again. Each time you are done, look around and spend a minute to be thankful for everything. Tell yourself you love yourself.

Exercise #4:
Take a shower and experience it. Don't think about anything else you did or have to do that day. Do

not judge how the shower feels or label it. Simply experience it, as if it was your very first shower. This is the essence of being present. It is your first time doing everything because if you appreciate reality and understand how everything changes, then it has to be your first time you are in this very moment. Since there are no guarantees in life, it may also be your last shower, so experience it fully. Take this same exercise out of the shower and into the kitchen where you will practice being present while you eat. Once you practice Exercises #3 and #4 enough, you will be able to become present whenever you want.

Exercise #5:
Watch the sky more. The sky is a metaphor for life, it is always changing. Take five minutes a day to watch the sunrise in the morning and five minutes to watch it set in the evening. Experience what you see fully. This exercise is not only an exercise in presence; it is an exercise in perspective. You will quickly feel how small you are in comparison to the Universe. This feeling is actually a feeling of freedom because your mind convinces you that you are more important than you are. We all need to be brought back into perspective with relation to the Universe and realize we may be small, but we are no smaller than anything else. The Universe

does not revolve around anyone, although some people truly believe that it does revolve around them. They are living in an illusion created by their own egos.

Occasionally, take time out on your way to work to pull over and watch the sunrise while you are practicing being present. Take note later how pulling over and watching the sunrise changes your whole day. I am sure you have heard people who have had near-death experiences say they now watch more sunsets and sunrises and eat more ice cream. This is because these are present-moment experiences where the senses are appreciated.

Exercise #6:
Love your inner child. Take the time to meditate, and imagine hugging yourself when you were younger and perhaps did not receive the love you deserved. Imagine a time when you accomplished something and did not get the love you deserved. Hug yourself, and give yourself the love and recognition you deserve.

Now, imagine forgiving yourself when you did something wrong. Imagine you are now the parent of your own inner child, and you are giving the child the love he or she deserves. Whenever you feel emotional pain, give yourself the love and/or forgiveness you deserve. I get a big knot in my stomach when I feel

117

emotional pain. That is a sign my inner child needs to be loved and nurtured. Take the time to do just that. Don't spoil your inner child with sympathy, food, or drugs, but give your inner child the true unconditional love he/she deserves.

Also, when you experience a positive intuitive moment from your spirit, take the time to praise and nurture your inner child for the experience. Listening to your intuition and encouraging it will, of course, bring out your spirit more often. It's time to quit blaming others, and it's time to be your own parent and best friend.

Exercise #7:
Learn to laugh at yourself and keep going. This doesn't mean you should be self-deprecating and cut yourself down. It just means that you shouldn't take yourself so seriously. It's all about keeping your perspective to keep going. Your ego and other egos will try to convince you to stop, but they cannot repress a spirit who is able to laugh at itself and keep going.

These are seven exercises to help you experience being present more often and help you keep your perspective in line with reality. You can do these exercises as your schedule permits. You must do them, though, or time will pass you by. That is what happens when you don't live in the present, time passes you by.

CHAPTER 13
BACK TO REALITY
- OR -
BACK TO THE ILLUSION

Iwent back to work six weeks after I got out of the hospital (part-time, at first) even though the doctor told me it would take three to six months. However, it took almost a year to fully recover. It felt like I got kicked in the head by a horse each day for the first two months. It took six months for my hair to come back and a little longer before my head felt stable and attached again.

I was happy, though. I spent a lot of time looking at the sky and watching the leaves blossom on the trees. I was in awe of nature and thankful I was able to experience nature through my senses.

During the recovery period, a few significant things happened. I was so happy to be alive, but I felt guilty for being so happy. I felt guilty for living. "Why did I get so lucky?" I kept asking myself. I kept thinking about people who were not as fortunate as I was.

What would people who went through something similar, but died, expect me to do?

Then one afternoon, as I fell asleep on my couch, I kept asking myself why I was so lucky. I had a dream. In the dream, a voice spoke to me. The voice represented all of those who died suddenly at young age. The voice said, "Be happy, be happy. It's all you owe us. It's your only obligation."

Happiness is not only your right, it is your obligation. When you sincerely appreciate the fact you are alive right now, it is impossible not to be happy right now.

Happiness is my obligation to those who were not as fortunate as I was. I knew I could be happy as long as I kept experiencing each moment to the fullest and kept thanking God for each experience, moment by moment, second by second. That's what I did, continuously. I was breathing, seeing, hearing, smelling, tasting, and touching everything as if it was my first time, and it could be my last because that was the reality of the situation.

I realized I might only live one year, or I might live five years, or I might live thirty years. I had to plan my life accordingly. If I was going to die in one year, I wanted to make sure I did everything I wanted to do in a year, but if it turned out that I lived longer than a year I had to make sure I didn't do anything crazy that would put me in jeopardy for the rest of my life. So, I decided I would do one thing each year, and I kept the idea a secret.

The power lies in keeping a secret, as I discussed in Lesson Unlearned #10. Less than two years after my operation, I took a new job and did not tell anyone at my new job about my operation.

I did things for me I never let myself do before. A year after my operation, I joined a singles club to have some fun. I went to Cancun, Mexico, twice and the Bahamas once. I developed some great friendships. I dated some beautiful women who were attracted to me simply because I was so happy. I even took a six-week, stand-up comedy class.

I didn't know where I got the idea to take a comedy class, but for some reason I had to take that comedy class. I took the class, and gave one stand-up comedy routine in front of an audience of one hundred people. It went well, even though I felt a lot of anxiety. I decided to quit after giving one performance because it was a great experience and a great memory. I wanted to keep it that way. Some people go through a mid-life crisis and jump out of an airplane and some people take a comedy class.

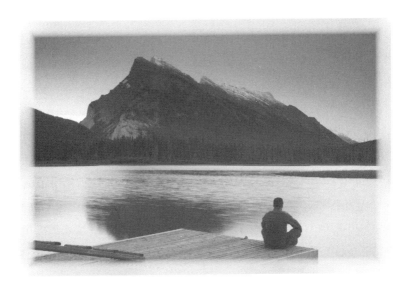

Lesson Unlearned #13
It's Your Secret

Write down one thing (only one thing) you would like to do if you had one year to live. There's only one hitch, there are no guarantees, so when making your choice, you have to consider you may live for five, ten, or more than thirty years. Just because you only have one year to live doesn't mean you should sell everything and hitchhike around the world, unless that's what you really want. Obviously, the one thing has to benefit you and it may benefit others.

What is your spirit telling you to do, but you're not listening? This is the year to listen.

Other than the one thing you want, your life continues as it is now. *You must not tell anyone, other than a close family member, you are living as if you only have one year to live. Keeping this secret gives you great power.*

You will continue to live your regular life, but throughout every day, ask yourself what would you do in this situation if you only had one year to live, even though you might live longer. This mind-set brings you immediately into the present moment. Which brings us to the other secret, don't forget to nurture your spirit with self-talk throughout the day and to wiggle your toes and fingers and smile to yourself without anyone else knowing why. Remember, it's your secret.

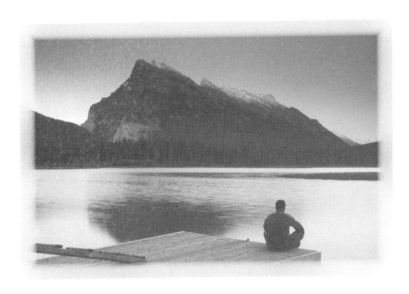

CHAPTER 14
THE ADDED BENEFIT

I had an MRI every quarter the first year after my operation. Then I had two MRIs in the second year and one a year after that. After five years, the surgeon said I didn't have to come back any more.

I had a lot of fun in my early forties. I told people it was my second childhood and that's how I lived. I was serious and quiet at work, but outside of work I had fun. When I made my promise years earlier to do the best with the cards I was dealt, I never, in my wildest dreams, thought I would have so much fun. After a while, though, I felt something was missing. I did not have a real purpose.

There must be some reason I am alive.

I wanted to give back, but I did not know how. Then, I utilized the same five principles I used to be happy after my operation, only I changed the third principle.

1. Develop an attitude of abundance.

2. Keep a big picture perspective.

3. Promise God I will find my purpose. I will do everything in my power to keep my promise.

4. Take little steps. Live in the present and concentrate fully on those little steps.

5. Don't forget to laugh.

I thought about volunteering at a local hospital or nursing home. I thought about turning my brain tumor story into a book, but I knew the story wasn't finished. Nothing seemed right. I decided to give up. Then on December 31, 2002, almost seven years after my operation, I made a New Year's resolution to join Toastmasters International. Toastmasters International is a non-profit organization that focuses on communication and leadership skills. I made the resolution to join Toastmasters for four reasons.

1. I would have something in common with my daughter. Alissa was seventeen at the time and on her way to becoming a finalist in high school state speech competition.

2. Maybe, after being in Toastmasters for ten years, I would have enough courage to tell people my story.

3. Maybe speaking in front of an audience would be fun even though the very thought of it made me anxious.

4. For some reason, I felt drawn to it as I was drawn to the comedy class five years earlier.

Joining Toastmasters was my 2003 New Year's resolution. I immediately got up enough courage to attend a meeting in June 2003.

I attended two meetings as a guest. I did not say a word during either meeting. My hands were sweating the whole time at the thought of having to say something. At the end of both meetings the person in charge asked me if I had any guest comments. I said no because I was too scared to talk and afraid of saying the wrong thing.

After the second meeting, I joined because I knew it was the only way I would push myself into speaking. After my first speech, my evaluator said I did a good job and my facial expressions matched what I was saying, but he said I needed to work on my gestures and vocal variety.

As the evaluator was talking, a voice in the back of my head said, "They teach people to talk with their hands." Then the voice yelled, "*YES!*" (with a fist pump).

As I drove home after my first speech, I had these thoughts. *I have spent my whole life trying to control my emotions and not talk with my hands. I can't believe they teach people to talk with their hands. I have no idea what my facial expressions look like, but in the past, people often said things to me like, "Why are you looking at me like that, and what's that look for?" I had been slapped several times in*

*my life for my facial expressions, but this was the first time
anyone said something positive about my facial expressions.*

I remembered my brother telling me I have the
quietest and the loudest voice he had ever heard.
*Hmm, if the people in Toastmasters want facial expressions,
gestures, and vocal variety, I will give them facial expressions,
gestures, and vocal variety.* I smiled all the way home.

I noticed a few people gave speeches about books
they had read. My second speech was a book report.
I took the cover off a book and pasted a picture of my
brain tumor to one of the pages inside of the book. *I
knew there was a reason I asked for a copy of my X-rays years
earlier.* I told the small audience in the Toastmasters
club the book was a story about the author who had a
brain tumor, and I showed the audience the picture of
the tumor in the book. I told them the author survived
and now he is really happy. At the end of the speech
I said, "Not only is this one of the best books I've ever
read, it's the only book I've ever written . . . Well I am
not done writing it yet."

All of the audience members dropped their jaws
and their eyes got real big.

I started getting more creative with my speeches
because I received so much positive feedback from my
first few speeches. I never knew I was creative. Then
again, I never knew my facial expressions, gestures,

and vocal variety were a good thing.

One woman told me I had talent. I was forty-nine years old. It was the first time in my life anyone had ever said I had talent. Another guy asked me if I had ever taken acting lessons. I said, "I've been acting my whole life, trying not to be like this."

I won the Toastmasters 2005 District 6 International Speech Contest with a speech about my brain tumor. District 6 primarily encompasses the state of Minnesota. After I won the contest, a guy came up to me and said, "You're not that good; I could have won if I had a brain tumor."

I said, "I'll pray for it to happen, if you will!" Well, I didn't actually say that, but I thought about it.

I practiced my brain tumor speech at several small Toastmasters clubs before I competed in the District level contest. One time when I finished my speech at a small club, a woman said, "That's a good story, but I think you made it up."

I said, "I have the picture, what more do you want?"

She said, "I don't care, I think you made it up."

I said, "OK."

A few minutes later, the same woman said, "I heard you are competing in the Tall Tales contest too. What is your Tall Tale about?"

I said, "It's just a little story about when my grandfather started Toastmasters." She asked, "Did he really?"

Arrrrrrh! God, she doesn't believe my real story, but she believes my Tall Tale. Arrrrrrh! I never in my wildest dreams believed I would have so much fun!

From the spring of 2005 through the spring of 2007, I placed in the top three (at the District level) in five different speech contests. Only one was about my brain tumor.

I tell you this story because, before my operation, I thought I was cursed with a bad personality I had to change. Remember the story in the preface about the girl who told me I had short choppy sentences like a second grader and the professor who said I had short concise sentences like Hemingway. My hope is you will not repress your spirit because of something negative someone said, or if you have already, it's not too late for your spirit to live and for you to find your purpose.

Remember, you cannot change your spirit. You can accept, acknowledge, and love your spirit, and you can hone your spirit with your conscious and subconscious mind to find and fulfill your purpose.

Lesson Unlearned #14
Finding Your Purpose

To discover your purpose, implement the five-step process.

1. Develop an attitude of abundance.

2. Keep a big picture perspective.

3. Promise yourself and God you will find your purpose. Do everything in your power to find your purpose and fulfill your promise.

4. Take little steps. Live in the present and concentrate fully on those little steps.

5. Don't forget to laugh.

Think about these questions until the answers come to you.

- What raw talent does your spirit have?

- How can you use this talent to make the world a better place?

- Do you have the passion to pay the price (remember price isn't always about money) to develop the raw talent your spirit possesses?

- Write down your biggest strengths.

- Write down your biggest weaknesses.

If I would have answered the previous questions before my operation, I would have written down that I only have one strength:

1. I am a hard worker. I am working real hard to change my personality so I don't have the weaknesses listed below.

I would have said my weaknesses include the following:

1. I don't always think before I speak.

2. Not everyone likes my quick witted sense of humor.

3. People don't like my facial expressions.

4. I talk with my hands.

5. I whisper sometimes. I yell most of the time.

The point is do not overlook the possibility that what you think are weaknesses are actually strengths you are covering up. I spent forty years working hard to change instead of accepting myself and figuring out where I could use my strengths and how I could hone them.

Once you have discovered your purpose, you can use the same five-step formula to develop and hone your spirit.

1. Develop an attitude of abundance.

2. Keep a big picture perspective.

3. Promise to do everything you can to sharpen your spirit.

4. Take little steps. Live in the present and concentrate fully on those little steps.

5. Don't forget to laugh.

You can use the five-step process to accomplish anything. You must want it bad enough to promise you will do everything in your power to get it and you must not forget the other steps.

Your purpose must help people and what you receive must be for your spirit and not for your ego. That is what makes it your purpose. By this, I mean your actions must be congruent with your spirit. Your purpose has to be something you really want to do and would do without praise, reward, or fear. You do it because it comes natural to you.

You cannot fail when you utilize the five-step process because of the following reasons:

1. The first two steps concentrate on being happy right now; therefore, there is no pressure to accomplish your goal. You are already happy.

2. Your long-term goal has been chosen by your spirit. This means you will have passion to keep following the path. A path chosen by your ego

will fade away because it is a means to an end, not the end. When your path is aligned with your spirit, the path and the process are the end. The only question is how far on the path you will go.

When you promise yourself you will do your best, you automatically picture the goal and concentrate on the current little steps you have to take. You take one day at a time and one small goal at a time. You focus your energy on what you can control.

Imagine two people walking across the desert. The first person is walking for competition. The first person tries to concentrate, but thoughts of winning, losing, pain, discomfort, and quitting creep into the mind.

Now imagine a second person walking across the desert who just survived a lion attack, but still has to walk across the desert. The second person is thankful to be alive. The second person has a vision of making it to safety on the other side of the desert, and concentrates on the steps it takes to get there.

The second person's focus is on appreciation, the goal, and what it takes to get there. The conscious mind, the subconscious mind, and the spirit are all in harmony. With this indomitable spirit, and mind-set there is no resistance. There is no resistance because the goal has been chosen by your conscious mind and your spirit. There is no resistance because there is no thought. There is only a picture of the goal in your mind and concentration on the present. There is a strong commitment to do your best and that is exactly what will happen.

Our spirit lives in the present. When another ego, or our own ego, criticizes our spirit, we have the tendency to repress our spirit by not living in the present. The spirit is replenished when we live in the present. If we take constructive feedback, we are encouraging ourselves to live in the present. Our spirit will be replenished and sharpened. Our spirit will become the best it can be.

Of course, it is unfortunately common for other egos and our own ego to offer destructive criticism to convince us to repress our spirit. Remember my example of when I told my dad I was at the top of my class out of eight hundred students and he said, "There must be a lot of stupid people going to that school." When a person's ego says something like that about your spirit, you must smile and say to yourself, "I accomplished something good and you cannot take that away from me. It's my self- esteem and you cannot have it." Keep your commitment to yourself, for that is part of loving yourself.

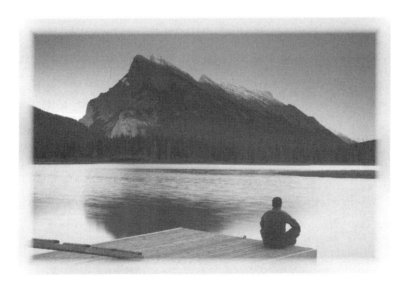

CHAPTER 15
And GOD Said, "HOW MANY TIMES DO I HAVE TO TELL YOU?"

On September 20 2005, nine years, seven months, and five days after my operation, I was canoeing with my brother, Steve, on a remote lake in northern Minnesota. We let the wind carry us down a long narrow lake, which was great until it was time to go back. We paddled hard, fighting against the wind and trying to stay close to shore. The wind blew the canoe sideways and away from the shoreline. We were perpendicular to the shoreline instead of parallel, and then a big wave came crashing up and over the canoe.

The canoe was capsized and I struggled for my life under the water. I am not a good swimmer. That's an overstatement. I cannot swim well at all, and I am very afraid of drowning.

My head popped up out of the water, and I grabbed the side of the canoe, which was full of water. I was clinging to the side of the canoe, and my brother was clinging to the other side. We lost everything we had except the canoe paddles and our life jackets, which we had on.

I tried to get back in the canoe while my brother tried to hold the canoe steady. The canoe was too full of water, and it was too windy. The canoe tipped over, and I went under the water again. When I came up out of the water, I grabbed the side of the canoe and said, "Steve, I don't know what we are going to do, but I am not going to do that again. Should we try to swim to shore?" I asked.

"No," Steve said, "we're supposed to stay with the canoe. I know that much."

"Good," I said, "because you can swim, and I can't. Steve, if we live, promise me you won't ever tell anyone about this."

"Roger, if we live, this would make a great speech."

"No way, Steve, no way am I ever going to tell anyone about this. They would just call us stupid. I would rather die right now than have anyone find out about this. I mean it, Steve. Promise me, you won't tell anyone about this."

"I promise I won't tell anyone, Roger."

Tipping the canoe over and being stranded in the middle of nowhere was different from the brain tumor because the brain tumor wasn't my fault, but this was clearly our fault and people would tease us and put us down for what happened.

We clung to the sides of the canoe like a couple of drowning rats hanging on for our lives. An hour went by, and we were still drifting down the middle of the long narrow lake instead of drifting to shore. We kept talking to each other, encouraging each other, and reminding each other what it would be like when we finally made it back to our car.

We drifted into shore one and a half hours after the canoe capsized. We were both shivering and on the verge of hypothermia. We took off our wet clothes, stripped to our underwear, paddled, and portaged back to our car. We reached our car six hours after tipping the canoe over. We each drank a gallon of water that night, and we were both fine the next day.

I did not tell anyone about this incident for several months because I was afraid of what people would say. Then it became clear to me: My spirit needs to express itself in an honest and truthful manner. This is what my spirit needs more than anything else. But my biggest fear is my fear of criticism and being called stupid for saying and doing the wrong thing.

This fear of criticism controlled my life and kept me from being myself. It was only because of my brain tumor experience that I was made aware of this fear.

Shortly after the canoe incident, I decided to become a professional speaker. I spent ten thousand dollars over the next year and a half on speech coaching to hone my craft. I am going to live the rest of my life helping and encouraging people to become the best they can be, and in doing so, I will be the best I can be.

I do have to ask for one favor from anyone who is reading this book. If you ever meet my brother, please don't tell him I told you the canoe story!

One day while I was finishing this book, I received an e-mail from a former co-worker whom I had not seen for ten years. This is what he wrote.

"Hey, Roger, I watched your video on your website, and it's very impressive. It's been a while since we have talked, but it struck me that you seem like an entirely different person. Pretty cool."

Lesson Unlearned #15
Be True to Yourself

Do you have the courage to show yourself to the world, I mean the real you? Do you have the honesty to discover your strengths? Do you have the character to develop those strengths to help others and fulfill your life purpose? Will you remember to laugh?

I used to think it was greedy when a super-rich person answered the question how much is enough money by saying, "Just a little more." I still think that is greedy but the truth is:

> *There are two kinds of people in this world:*
> *those who move forward*
> *and those who don't.*
> *No matter what your situation is*
> *You must be the kind of person who moves forward.*

At the time of this writing, I am fifty-three years old. Lately, I think a lot about my paternal grandmother. I never met my paternal grandmother. All I know about her is this: She came to the United States by herself when she was fifteen years old. Along with my grandfather, she raised eleven children. She was not educated, but she was a midwife and she delivered over one hundred babies.

I do not have any grandchildren yet, but if I ever do, I know they will think of me long after I am gone and they are in their fifties. I want them to say, "My grandfather did not even get started until he turned fifty. He gave speeches to help people. He talked about never quitting and never giving up." That's what I want my grandchildren to say about me.

What do you want people to remember about you? You have the opportunity today to create the life your spirit is craving. Go over the Lessons Unlearned and unlearn a few lessons that are holding you back. Be present. Love, nurture, and hone your inner child. Be true to yourself, fulfill your purpose, and don't forget to laugh.

There is only one exercise left. You are now ready for the Inspirational Challenge.

The Inspirational Challenge

1. Accept and love your self for who you are.

2. Identify a worthy goal and keep it private.

3. Concentrate on what you can control, so you can move forward.

4. Choose your path and continuously take small steps outside of your comfort zone, so you can become your best.

5. Never allow anyone to steal your self-esteem by belittling your accomplishments. Smile and remember they are trying to steal your self-esteem because their self-esteem is low.

6. Invite others, who say you are an inspiration to them, to embrace the Inspirational Challenge by giving them a copy of this page. Only give a copy of this Inspirational Challenge to someone who says you are an inspiration to them because the ultimate goal is to become an inspiration to others.

May you reach all of your goals and, more importantly, may you become an inspiration to all of those around you.

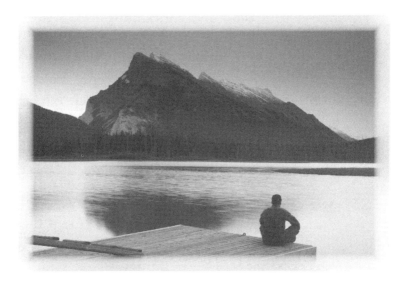

Acknowledgements

Thank you to all of the people who have supported me in my life and in the writing of this book. Thanks to all of the doctors and nurses who helped me and to all people who help other people. Thanks to Toastmasters International for allowing me to find my purpose and hone my spirit. Thanks to my editor and publisher, Sharron and Harry Stockhausen for your guidance and patience while I wrote this book. Thanks to my close buddies Greg, Wayne, Todd, and Dave for your humor and friendship throughout the writing process. Thanks to my friend Bonnie for leading the way and setting an example for me to follow. Thanks to my mother, Irene; sister, Linda; and brother, Steve, for understanding why I needed to write this book. Thanks to my daughter, Alissa, for being my inspiration.

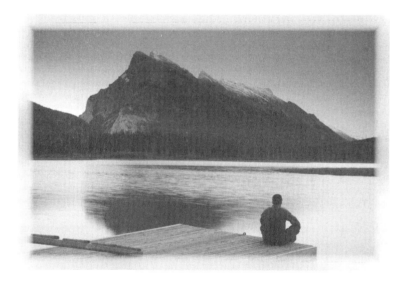

About the Author

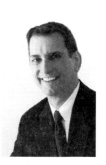

Roger Revak has had a variety of careers. He served four years in the US Air Force, eight years working in an iron ore mine, and eighteen years working in commercial banking, including the position of vice president.

When Roger was thirty years old, he was laid off from his blue-collar job in the iron ore mine at the same time his daughter was born. When he was thirty-four years old, he graduated from college Magna Cum Laude with a double major in accounting and finance. When he was forty years old, he learned he had a large brain tumor.

Determined to share what he learned from his experience with others, Roger joined Toastmasters and placed in the top three in five state-level Toastmasters speech contests.

Roger Revak is a professional speaker who shows individuals and organizations how to turn a difficult situation into a positive one.

Roger Revak lives in St. Paul, MN. You can visit him at www.rogerrevak.com and reach him at info@ rogerrevak.com.